THE ABR HANDBOOK:
AUDITORY BRAINSTEM RESPONSE

THE ABR HANDBOOK:
AUDITORY BRAINSTEM RESPONSE

Second Edition

Michael E. Glasscock III, M.D., F.A.C.S.
C. Gary Jackson, M.D., F.A.C.S.
Anne Forrest Josey, M.S., C.C.C.A.

All of the Otology Group
Nashville, Tennessee

1987
Thieme Medical Publishers, Inc., New York
Georg Thieme Verlag, Stuttgart · New York

Thieme Medical Publishers, Inc.
381 Park Avenue South
New York, New York 10016

Cover design: Wendy Ann Fredericks

The ABR Handbook:
Auditory Brainstem Response
Michael E. Glasscock III
C. Gary Jackson
Anne Forrest Josey

Library of Congress Cataloging in Publication Data

Glasscock, Michael E., 1933–
  The ABR handbook.
  Rev. ed. of: Brain stem electric response audiometery. 1981.
  Includes bibliographies and index.
  1. Audiometry, Evoked response. I. Jackson,
C. Gary. II. Josey, Anne Forrest. III. Glasscock, Michael E., 1933–   . Brain stem electric
response audiometry. IV. Title. V. Title: Auditory brainstem response. [DNLM: 1. Audiometry. 2. Audiometry,   Evoked   Response.
3. Brain   Stem—physiology. 4. Electrophysiology.
WV 272 G549b]
RF294.5.E87G57 1987   617.8'07547   86-30007

Typeset by Maple-Vail Book Mfg. Group, Binghamton, NY, U.S.A.
Printed and bound by R. R. Donnelley & Sons, Harrisonburg, VA, U.S.A.
Printed in the United States of America.

TMP ISBN 0-86577-202-9
GTV ISBN 3-13-599502-1

PREFACE TO THE SECOND EDITION

The second edition of our brainstem book was undertaken to update and expand current applications of ABR. Some of the text simply needed addition of state-of-the-art techniques, while other considerations required additional chapters.

Although use of the early auditory potentials has become widespread, there is still no consensus on nomenclature. However, many clinicians seem comfortable with ABR (Auditory Brainstem Response), and this explains the authors' update on terminology in this edition.

The second chapter was expanded to provide more physiologic information as background for interpretation. The technical and applications chapters were updated to include new information on ABR in the operating room.

An additional chapter was included to provide more extensive case material to put the ABR in perspective with total patient evaluation.

Since the use of the ABR is rapidly spreading and expanding, the authors look forward to further change and improvement in the future.

Michael E. Glasscock III
C. Gary Jackson
Anne Forrest Josey

PREFACE TO THE FIRST EDITION

This book is not meant to be a treatise on brain stem electric response audiometry (BERA), nor is it a reference work. It was written as a practical introduction to the clinical use of BERA for audiology students, residents, and practicing otolaryngologists. The Ph.D. audiologist with prior knowledge of BERA will not find this book intellectually stimulating.

We have attempted to standardize terminology as much as possible. This has been difficult to accomplish because the field is new and constantly changing. In some instances we have decided upon a term even though we realize that within a few months it might change. A prime example is the book's title, *Brain Stem Electric Response Audiometry*. Terminology for this procedure has shifted back and forth for the past two to three years. At present there is a move to use "Auditory Evoked Response Audiometry" which doubtless will spawn a new acronym, AERA. Although parts of this book may be dated by the time of publication, our intention is to provide an introduction to the subject as it relates to clinical practice. In this light, the book should serve its purpose for several years.

A section of test equipment was purposely omitted owing to the constant evolution of new equipment rendering each piece of hardware obsolete within two to three years of its manufacture. The underlying principles of neurophysiology and test methodology are less changeable, so that if one masters the test procedure on today's equipment, the knowledge can be easily transferred to the more sophisticated units of the future.

Above all, this book is clinically oriented, having been written with the clinical audiologist and the practicing otolaryngologist in mind. Its two sections deal with basic considerations (Chapters 1, 2, and 3) with clinical applications (Chapters 4 and 5). This arrangement should allow the individual to select an entry point for reading based upon his prior knowledge of BERA and what he wishes to obtain from the book.

This is not a cookbook on how to do BERA: the reader will not become proficient in performing and interpreting BERA tracings from this book. Rather, those who survive a reading of the book should have a solid working knowledge of BERA and its clinical applications. For technical proficiency in administering BERA, enrollment in one of the basic courses offered through the year is necessary.

CONTENTS

CHAPTER ONE

AN INTRODUCTION TO BRAINSTEM AUDIOMETRY

HISTORY

As auditory brainstem response (ABR) audiometry assumes its position as an important diagnostic procedure, it is appropriate to review the major events leading to its widespread use in clinical audiometry. A glossary of pertinent terms and classifications follows our historical account. Our review is intended only as a preface to the clinical chapters of this book. The reader is referred elsewhere for more detail.[1-4]

The origins of ABR can be traced to the animal experiments of the 19th century. In 1875, Caton[5] first reported that there was electrical activity in the brain, which could be demonstrated by evoked potentials in the rabbit. He was also the first to notice the unexpected spontaneous oscilations of the baseline that were later to become known as the electrocorticogram.

Danilevsky,[6] working in Russia, studied the spontaneous electrical activity of the brain in dogs in or around 1877. Essentially, he rediscovered evoked potentials in the dog rather than in the rabbit. Unlike Caton, he was aware of the auditory potentials. Between 1883 and 1891 Fleischl von Marxow,[7] Beck,[8] and Gotch and Horsley[9] actively pursued the recording of electrical activity of the brain in a variety of experimental animals, but it was Pravdich-Neminsky[10] who in 1913 first photographed the record of an animal electroencephalogram with a string galvanometer.

Until more sophisticated equipment was designed, researchers were limited in their range of activity. In the early part of the 20th century, electrophysiologists were working under very primitive conditions owing to the lack of sophisticated equipment. It was not until 1920 that an electrical amplifier was used in a physiological experiment by Forbes and Thacher;[11] the cathode-ray oscilloscope was not in general use until 1922. In the 1930s, oscilloscopic images were made bright enough and electrical amplifiers were stable enough to allow neurophysiologists to devote their time to experiments rather than to equipment problems.

In 1927, Forbes, Miller, and O'Connor[12] presented a series of rapidly repeated clicks to a cat's ear and were able to record the volley of

1

nerve impulses. Wever and Bray[13] performed a series of experiments that led to the development of the cochlear microphonic 2 years later by Saul and Davis.[14] Wever and his associate listened to words spoken into a cat's ear that had been recorded and fed into a telephone receiver. To their amazement, the words were intelligible!

By 1935, Derbyshire and Davis[15] had established the hair cells of the organ of Corti as the generator of the cochlear microphonic. Their work was published as a definitive study of the action potentials in the auditory nerve. Four years later a microintracellular electrode was developed by Hodgkin and Huxley[16] to record the membrane potential and the action potential of the giant axon of the squid. In 1943, Galambos and Davis[17] reported the first response areas and characteristic frequencies of auditory units in the cat. Tasaki[18] was responsible for penetrating the first-order fibers of the cochlear nerve in the guinea pig. Kiang,[19] by use of micromanipulators and computers, obtained discharge patterns in single fibers in the cat auditory nerve in 1965.

By the early 1960s, neurophysiologists were beginning to record evoked auditory potentials. The groundwork for their studies had been laid by the early investigators of the human electroencephalogram (EEG). The alpha rhythm was first demonstrated by Berger[20] in 1929. Loomis (as referenced in Davis),[4] working independently, rediscovered the EEG and was responsible for naming the "K" complex in 1935. By 1954, Dawson[21] was able to use the first electronic response averager, an analogue device with 124 time points and a mechanical revolving commutator to charge each condenser in turn. The response averager was employed in the recording of the slow somatosensory cortical responses to electrical stimulation of the ulnar nerve in the human. By 1961, Davis[4] had acquired a digital computer and began using it extensively in his electrophysiology experiments.

Subsequently, in 1963, the New York Academy of Arts and Sciences announced a symposium that brought together investigators in the various fields of averaged potentials, including visual, somatosensory, auditory, myogenic, and neurogenic. The following year a program was presented in Toronto concerning the identification and management of the young deaf child by use of electric response audiometry. Because of the widening interest and expanding knowledge of the subject of evoked potentials, the International Electric Response Audiometry Study Group was founded in 1968.

By 1968, slow cortical response audiometry under sedation was being attempted in some centers; however, it proved to be unreliable in a clinical setting and never gained widespread acceptance. At the same time, Yoshie and associates,[22] Aran and LeBert,[23] and Sohmer and Feinmesser[24] applied the technique of response averaging to the ear and introduced electrocochleography (ECochG). Because of the need to place an electrode directly on the basal coil of the cochlea, this procedure never gained wide acceptance in the United States. Sohmer and Feinmesser were able to use "far field" electrodes to perform ECochG by placing the active electrode in the ear canal rather than through the tympanic membrane and on to the cochlea. By 1971, Jewett and Williston[25] had established a definitive description of ABR, and in 1974 Hecox and Galambos[26] expanded this definition to the audiometry of infants and adults. From 1974 to the present time there have been numerous contributors to the clinical use of ABR. Starr and Hamilton[27] are renowned for their description of the possible origins of waves I through V and for having demonstrated the value of ABR in the diagnosis of central nervous system disease. Selters and Brackmann,[28] as well as House and Brackmann,[29] Glasscock and associates,[30] and Josey, Glasscock, and Jackson[31] have shown that ABR is highly reliable in the demonstration of cerebellopontine angle lesions such as acoustic tumors.

With the widespread use of ABR in a clinical setting, equipment manufacturers have made a concerted effort to simplify and modernize their products. Throughout the country, courses in the practical use of ABR are presented, and there is little question that this diagnostic procedure has established for itself a permanent position in the modern evaluation scheme of the auditory system. The cumbersome, experimental recording of evoked auditory potentials has moved from the laboratory into the audiology clinic, where it is now a practical diagnostic study.

GLOSSARY

Classification of Auditory Evoked Potentials

Of the many different electric responses to auditory stimuli, most arise in the central nervous system, some are generated in the cochlea, and still others are reflex responses in muscles. In order to discuss ABR it is important to understand the nomenclature. Therefore, the following terms set forth by the London Symposium of the International Electric Response Audiometry Study Group (1975) are presented.

Evoked Potentials and Electric Responses

By definition a response is evoked. Thus, "evoked response" is somewhat redundant. Potentials are evoked; therefore, evoked potential and electric response are proper designations.

Anatomical Terminology

On the basis of electrode placement, the first distinction among auditory evoked potentials is anatomic: "at the vertex" or "in the ear." In the first subdivision, one or two reference electrodes are placed in the earlobe or mastoid while the active electrode is attached to the top of the head or vertex. Vertex (V) potentials measured in this fashion are classified by latency as fast, middle, slow, or late. This method of recording evoked potentials is called "far field" technique.

The second subdivision is referred to as ECochG. The reference electrodes are placed on the earlobe and the active electrode is placed within the middle ear or external auditory canal. If classified by latency (as with the V potentials), these evoked potentials would be referred to as early potentials.

Physiologic Terminology

The second distinction among evoked potentials is physiologic and is based on whether the potential is continuing (alternating current [AC]) or sustained (direct current [DC]). The continuing potentials have been assigned specific names and abbreviations.

Cochlear Microphonic (CM).   A continuing AC response generated chiefly by the external hair cells in the organ of Corti.

Summating Potential (SP).   A continuing DC response generated in both internal and external hair systems, depending on whether it is negative or positive.

Frequency Following Response (FFR).   A continuing AC response generated in several nuclei of the brainstem.

Sustained Cortical Potential (SCP).   A continuing DC response generated in the cerebral (auditory) cortex.

Contingent Negative Variant (CNV).   A very late DC shift developing in certain situations between a warning signal and an expected imperative stimulus.

Latency Terminology

The on-effect responses are subdivided on the basis of their latencies as to fast, middle, slow, or late. A particular wave is designated by P if it is vertex-positive and by N if it is vertex-negative. A subscript is used to give the on-effects' most characteristic latency in a normal hearing adult well above threshold level, for instance at a sensation level of 60 decibels (dB). For example, a late cortex wave would be designated P_{300}.

Latency responses have generally been categorized as follows:

1.   *Early* (occurring in the first 5 milliseconds [msec] after stimulation). The action potential is generally the auditory response analyzed in this time base and represents cochlear activity as it is conducted through the eighth nerve.

2.   *Fast* (occurring 2 to 12 msec after stimulation). The auditory brainstem response, the Jewett sequence of six to seven waves, is the potential most often recorded in this time category. These wavelets are generally assigned roman numerals according to the Jewett[25] classification. Wave V, the most prominent event, occurs at about 6 msec at suprathreshold intensity. The responses represent eighth nerve and brainstem activity.

A somewhat longer response, generated at this same level, is called the slow-wave component of the brainstem response or SWR (Klein).[32] It occurs at 12 msec after stimulation at well above threshold intensity and at about 20 msec near threshold and is used to track thresholds by frequency in audiologic applications.

3. *Middle* (occurring 12 to 50 msec after stimulation). These responses are thought to include both sonomotor and neurogenic responses arising from the cortex. The response occurring at 30 to 35 msec, often labelled P_{35}, is the most useful of these variants.

4. *Slow* (occurring 50 to 300 msec after stimulation). This response has a vertex-positive peak at about 180 msec and vertex-negative peaks at 90 and 250 msec.

5. *Late* (occurring 250 to 600 msec after stimulation). These cortical responses include information about the neuropsychology of hearing and listening. One series used clinically is designated P_{300} because the predominant suprathreshold peak occurs at 300 msec post-stimulation. Another frequently used pattern in this time base is the CNV.

The ABR

The ABR has applications in both neurotologic and audiologic evaluations. These responses vary from those of a normal subject according to the nature of the pathology and the degree of loss of sensitivity. Because of its considerable clinical utility, it is the focus of this book.

This fast response series occurs in the first 10 to 12 msec after stimulation. In the literature the wavelets are often labelled with roman numerals, after the convention of Jewett.[25] The peaks in this sequence are generally named for their vertex-positive peaks, represented in the upward direction in this book. (Some articles, especially in the European literature, reflect positivity downward.) The ABR profiles synchronous discharge to an appropriate stimulus at threshold and suprathreshold levels. The level of brain activity monitored by the ABR is primitive and includes the auditory periphery, the eighth nerve and, in part, the brainstem. This averaged evoked potential to sound is a series of wavelets (Jewett and Williston[25]), which are visible as a result of time-locked averaging after stimulation. There are five to seven waves in a normal subject occurring at 1 msec intervals beginning at about 1.5 to 2 msec. The normal ABR pattern is illustrated in Figure 1–1. Factors affecting the acquisition of the response and pathologic findings in these patterns will be discussed in detail in Chapters 3 and 4.

There are two general categories of application of these responses. One reason for obtaining them may be as part of a neurodiagnostic evaluation. In this application, the clinician compares the waveform or morphology and latencies of the peaks to normal responses. For example, a peak which occurs later than normal could suggest a pathologic condition at some point or points in the region these responses are generated, from

Figure 1–1. Example of normal ABR recording. (Recorded from a 23 year old man with normal hearing. Click stimulus at 75 dB nHL, 2000 samples.)

the inner ear through the brainstem. These site-of-lesion applications will be outlined in Chapter 5.

A second use of ABR is in the determination of threshold. Within certain limits, ABR can provide information about the sensitivity of the peripheral mechanism. In special cases, such as an infant at risk for hearing loss, ABR can provide a quick, reliable assessment without discomfort to the patient. Examples of such applications are described in Chapter 5.

Although this book describes many useful applications of ABR in neuroaudiologic evaluation, there is certainly no intention of suggesting its use as the best or only neuroaudiologic tool. Test battery integration will be illustrated in the case examples in Chapter 6.

REFERENCES

1. Brazier, M. A. B.: The historical development of neurophysiology, in Field, J., Magoun, H. W., Hall, V. E. (eds.): *Handbooks of Physiology, Section 1: Neurophysiology.* Washington, D.C., American Physiological Society, 1959, vol. 1, chap. 1.
2. Brazier, M. A. B.: *A History of the Electrical Activity of the Brain.* New York, The Macmillan Co., 1961.
3. Neff, W. D., and Keidel, W. D. (eds.): *Handbook of Sensory Physiology.* Berlin, Heidelberg, New York, Springer-Verlag, 1974, vol V/2.
4. Davis, H.: Principles of electric response audiometry. Ann Otol Rhinol Laryngol 85 (Suppl 28):1–96, 1976.
5. Caton, R.: The electric currents of the brain. Br Med J 2:278, 1875.
6. Danilevsky, V. Y.: Investigations into the physiology of the brain. Thesis, University of Karkov, 1877.
7. Fleischl von Marxow, E.: Mittheilung betreffend die Physiologie der Hirnrinde. Zbl Physiol 4:538, 1890.
8. Beck, A.: Die Bestimmung der Localisation der Gehirn—und Rückenmarkfunctionen vermittelst der electrischen Erscheinungen. Cbl Physiol 4:473–476, 1890.
9. Gotch, F., and Horsley, V.: Über den Gebrauch der Elektricität für die Lokalisierung der Erregungserscheinungen im Centralnervensystem. Zbl Physiol 4:649–651, 1891.

10. Pravdich-Neminsky, V. V.: Ein Versuch der Registrierung der elektrischen Gehirnerscheinungen. Zbl Physiol 27:951–960, 1913.
11. Forbes, A., and Thacher, C.: Amplification of action currents with the electron tube in recording with the string galvanometer. Am J Physiol 52:409–471, 1920.
12. Forbes, A., Miller, R. H., and O'Connor, J.: Electric responses to acoustic stimuli in the decerebrate animal. Am J Physiol 80:363–380, 1927.
13. Wever, E. G., and Bray, C. W.: The nature of acoustic response: The relation between sound frequency and frequency of impulses in the auditory nerve. J Exp Psychol 13:373–387, 1930.
14. Saul, L. J., and Davis, H.: Action currents in the central nervous system: I. Action currents of the auditory tracts. Arch New Psychiatr 28:1104–1116, 1932.
15. Derbyshire, A. J., and Davis, H.: The action potentials of the auditory nerve. Am J Physiol 113:476–504, 1935.
16. Hodgkin, A. L., and Huxley, A. F.: Action potentials recorded from inside a nerve fiber. Nature 144:710–711, 1939.
17. Galambos, R., and Davis, H.: The response of single auditory-nerve fibers to acoustic stimulation. J Neurophysiol 6:39–57, 1943.
18. Tasaki, I.: Nerve impulses in individual auditory nerve fibers of guinea pig. J. Neurophysiol 17:97–122, 1954.
19. Kiang, NY-S: *Discharge Patterns of Single Fiber in the Cat's Auditory Nerve.* Cambridge, MIT Press, 1965.
20. Berger, H.: Uber das Elektrenkephalogramm des Menschen. I. Arch f Psychiatr 87:527–570, 1929.
21. Dawson, G. D.: A summation technique for the detection of small evoked potentials. Electroencephalogr Clin Neurophysiol 6:65–84, 1954.
22. Yoshie N., Ohashi, T., and Suzuki, T.: Nonsurgical recording of auditory nerve action potentials in man. Laryngoscope 77:76–85, 1967.
23. Aran, J. M., and LeBert, G.: Les responses nerveuses cochleaeres chez l'homme, image du fonctionnement de l'oreille et nouveau test d'audiometrie objective. Rev Laryngol Otol Rhinol (Bord) 89:361–378, 1968.
24. Sohmer, H., and Feinmesser, M.: Cochlear action potentials recorded from the external ear in man. Ann Otol Rhinol Laryngol 76:427–435, 1967.
25. Jewett, D. L., and Williston, J. S.: Auditory evoked far-fields averaged from the scalp of humans. Brain 94:681–696, 1971.
26. Hecox, K., and Galambos, R.: Brain stem auditory evoked responses in human infants and adults. Arch Otolaryngol 99:30–33, 1974.
27. Starr, A., and Hamilton, A.: Correlation between confirmed sites of neurological lesions of far-field auditory brain stem responses. Electroencephalogr Clin Neurophysiol 41:595–608, 1976.
28. Selters, W. A., and Brackmann, D. E.: Acoustic tumor detection with brain stem electric response audiometry. Arch Otolaryngol 103:181–187, 1977.
29. House, J. W., and Brackmann, D. E.: Brain stem audiometry in neurotologic diagnosis. Arch Otolaryngol 105:305, 1979.
30. Glasscock, M. E., Jackson, C. G., Josey, A. F., Dickins, J. R., and Wiet, R. J.: Brain stem evoked response audiometry in a clinical practice. Laryngoscope 89:1021–1034, 1979.
31. Josey, A. F., Glasscock, M. E. and Jackson, C. G.: Auditory brainstem response patterns in eighth nerve tumors. Presented at the American Speech-Language Hearing Association convention, San Francisco, Nov. 1984.
32. Klein, A. J.: Properties of the brain-stem response slow-wave component. Arch Otolaryngol 109:6–12, 1983.

CHAPTER TWO

THE AUDITORY SYSTEM

This chapter provides a synopsis of the anatomy and physiology of the auditory system as a basis for our discussion of auditory brainstem response (ABR) methodology and clinical application. The reader is referred to the following publications for more detail: the anatomy of the outer, middle, and inner ear is particularly well covered in *Gray's Anatomy*,[1] the detailed structure of the cochlea and the central pathways of the auditory system can be found in Schuknecht's *Pathology of the Ear*,[2] and the physiology of the auditory system has been described extensively by Davis.[3]

ANATOMY OF THE AUDITORY SYSTEM

The auditory system consists of the outer, middle, and inner ear, the cochlear nerve, the cochlear nuclei, the brainstem pathways, and the auditory cortex.

The Outer Ear

The outer ear consists of the auricle (pinna) and the external auditory canal. The auricle is an ovoid structure, with its larger portion located superiorly. The lateral surface is concave, having numerous depressions and protrusions, each assigned a specific name. The auricle consists of one large piece of cartilage covered by thin skin closely adherent to the cartilage and continuous with the epithelium of the external auditory meatus. The vascular supply is from the posterior branch of the external carotid artery, the superficial temporal artery, and the occipital artery.

The sensory nerves are the great auricular (cervical plexus), the auricular branch of the vagus, the auriculotemporal branch of the mandibular (V-3), and the lesser occipital (cervical plexus) (Fig. 2–1).

The external canal is two-thirds bone and one-third cartilage. The skin is thin and closely adherent to the underlying structures. The overall length is approximately 2.5 centimeters (cm), with the cerumen glands

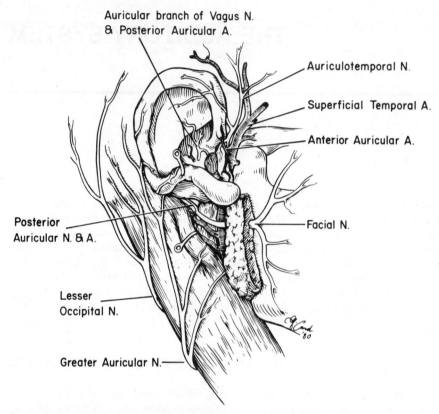

Auricular branch of Vagus N.
& Posterior Auricular A.

Auriculotemporal N.

Superficial Temporal A.

Anterior Auricular A.

Posterior
Auricular N. & A.

Facial N.

Lesser
Occipital N.

Greater Auricular N.

Figure 2–1. The sensory nerves are the great auricular (cervical plexus), auricular branch of the vagus, auriculotemporal branch of the mandibular (V-3), and the lesser occipital (cervical plexus).

located in the outer one-third of the canal and placed superiorly. The junction of the cartilaginous and bony canals is referred to as the isthmus. The cartilage of the canal is deficient anteriorly, where two-thirds of the fissures are present. The bony canal is narrower than the cartilaginous portion and terminates medially at the tympanic sulcus. This V-shaped or grooved portion receives the fibrous anulus of the tympanic membrane. The sulcus is deficient superiorly in the area known as the notch of Rivinus.

Anterior to the bony canal lies the temporomandibular joint, and posterior to it are the mastoid air cells. The arteries supplying the external canal derive from the posterior auricular, internal maxillary, and temporal arteries. The external canal is innervated by the auriculotemporal branch of the mandibular nerve (V-3) and the auricular branch of the vagus.

The Middle Ear

The middle ear comprises the tympanic cavity, the eustachian tube, the tympanic membrane, and the ossicles.

Tympanic Membrane

The tympanic membrane closes the medial end of the external auditory canal. It has three distinct layers. The middle layer consists of interlacing collagenous fibers radiating away from the handle of the malleus (first ossicle), and the circumference of the membrane forms a thick ring (fibrous anulus) that rests in the tympanic sulcus of the bony external auditory canal. The outer surface of this fibrous middle layer is covered by skin that is continuous with the ear canal, but that does not contain rete pegs. The inner surface of the fibrous layer is covered with a mucous membrane that is continuous with that of the middle ear (Fig. 2–2).

The tympanic membrane is semitransparent, and the portion containing the fibrous layer is referred to as the pars tensa. A small triangular area of the drum lying superior to the short process of the malleus is known as the pars flacida or Schrapnell's membrane. Two fibrous folds

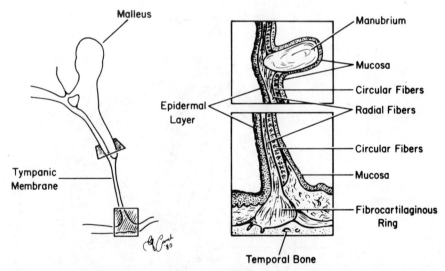

Figure 2–2. The tympanic membrane closes the medial end of the external auditory canal. It has three distinct layers. The middle layer consists of interlacing collagenous fibers radiating away from the handle of the malleus (first ossicle), and the circumference of the membrane forms a thick ring (fibrous anulus) that rests in the tympanic sulcus of the bony external auditory canal. The outer surface of this fibrous middle layer is covered by skin which is continuous with the ear canal, but which does not contain rete pegs. The inner surface of the fibrous layer is covered with mucous membrane which is continuous with that of the middle ear.

extending from the malleus to the edge of the notch of Rivinus are the anterior and posterior malleolar ligaments.

The tympanic membrane is cone-shaped, the most depressed part of the concavity or umbo corresponding to the tip of the handle of the malleus.

The main vascular supply enters the tympanic membrane superiorly and is derived from the internal maxillary artery. Additional vascularity comes from the postauricular and tympanic arteries (Fig. 2–3).

The eardrum is innervated by the auriculotemporal branch of the mandibular nerve, the auricular branch of the vagus nerve, and the tympanic branch of the glossopharyngeal nerve.

Tympanic Cavity

The middle ear or tympanic cavity is an irregular air-filled space lying within the temporal bone. The area just medial to the tympanic membrane is the tympanic cavity, whereas the space above the membrane is the epitympanic recess or attic. This space contains the head of the malleus and the body of the incus. Measuring from the attic to the floor of the

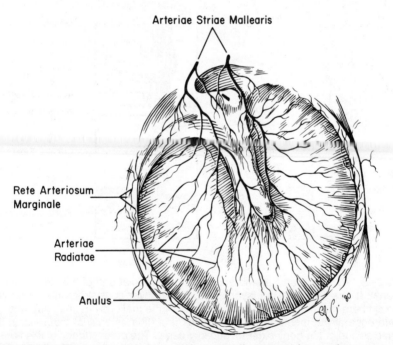

Arteriae Striae Mallearis

Rete Arteriosum
Marginale

Arteriae
Radiatae

Anulus

Figure 2–3. The main vascular supply enters the tympanic membrane superiorly and is derived from the internal maxillary artery. Additional vascularity comes from the postauricular and tympanic arteries.

middle ear cavity (hypotympanicum) and from the anterior to the posterior, the space is approximately 15 × 15 millimeters (mm). The transverse diameter measures 6 mm in the attic and 4 mm in the hypotympanicum. Just medial to the umbo, the space is only 2 mm wide (Fig. 2–4).

The roof of the tympanic cavity is called the tegmen tympani and consists of the thin layer of bone separating the attic from the dura overlying the temporal lobe. The floor or hypotympanicum consists of air cells similar to those found in the mastoid. The inferior aspect of this cell system consists of a thin layer of bone separating it from the dome of the jugular bulb. Posteriorly, the tympanic cavity communicates with the antrum of the mastoid and anteriorly with the eustachian or auditory tube, which connects the cavity to the nasopharynx. The bony portion is ap-

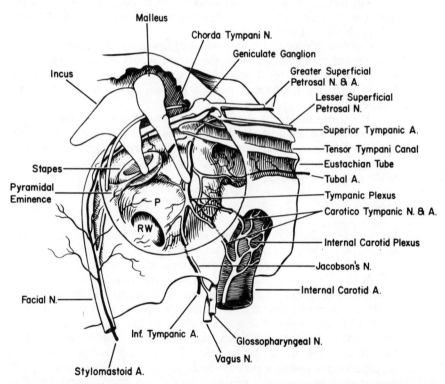

Figure 2–4. The middle ear or tympanic cavity is an irregular air-filled space lying within the temporal bone. The area just medial to the tympanic membrane is the tympanic cavity. The space above the membrane is the epitympanic recess or attic. This space contains the head of the malleus and body of the incus. Measuring from the attic to the floor of the middle ear cavity (hypotympanicum) and from anterior to posterior, the space is approximately 15×15 mm. The transverse diameter measures 6 mm in the attic and 4 mm in the hypotympanicum. Just medial to the umbo, the space is only 2 mm wide.

proximately one-third its length, the remaining two-thirds being cartila-ginous. The bony cartilaginous junction is known as the isthmus. As the tube enters the nasopharynx, there is an elevation of cartilage just poste-rior to the orifice called the torus tabaris. Behind this structure is a depression referred to as Rosenmüller's fossa. The mucous membrane of the middle ear cavity and the eustachian tube is respiratory in nature and contains cilia.

Just inferior to the eustachian tube and anterior to the lower half of the tympanic cavity lies the carotid canal containing the internal carotid artery.

The medial wall of the middle ear space comprises the basal coil of the cochlea (auditory portion of the inner ear) and is known as the pro-montory.

The fenestra vestibuli (oval window) opens into the vestibule of the inner ear. Its greatest diameter is in the horizontal plane. The third ossicle (stapes) lies in the oval window.

The fenestra cochlea (round window) lies below and behind the oval window and communicates with the scala tympani of the cochlea. It is closed by a three-layered secondary membrane (round window mem-brane) separating the fluid-filled scala tympani of the cochlea from the middle ear cavity.

The semicanal of the tensor tympani muscle, as well as the horizon-tal or middle ear segment of the facial nerve canal, are prominent projec-tions from the medial wall into the cavity. The second middle ear muscle, the stapedius, protrudes from the pyramidal eminence, where it attaches to the neck of the stapes.

Ossicles

The ossicles themselves are known as the malleus, incus, and stapes. The malleus has a head, neck, short or lateral process, and a handle that is buried within the fibrous layer of the tympanic membrane. The incus has a body, long and short processes, and an articular surface that interlocks with the head of the malleus. The lenticular process of the incus is a small, cartilaginous structure connecting the long process of the incus to the head of the stapes. The stapes itself looks like the stirrup of an En-glish saddle. The footplate lies in the oval window and is held in place by a fibrous ring, the anular ligament. Two crura or arches extend from the anterior and posterior portions of the footplate, forming the neck. The capitulum or head of the stapes rests on the neck and is covered by car-tilage. The malleus and incus are suspended in the attic by ligaments that allow them to vibrate as a unit.

The facial nerve passes through the middle ear and mastoid in the fallopian canal. In its mastoid segment, the facial nerve gives off the chorda tympani nerve, which transverses the tympanic cavity and exits through the iter chordae anterius and the petrotympanic fissure to supply taste to the anterior two-thirds of the tongue.

Vascular supply of the tympanic cavity is by way of the inferior tympanic artery, which is a branch of the ascending pharyngeal artery from the external carotid artery. The caroticotympanic branches of the internal carotid artery, the stylomastoid branch of the postauricular artery, and the tympanic branch of the internal maxillary artery also contribute to the vascular supply of the tympanic cavity.

The tympanic branch of the glossopharyngeal nerve (Jacobson's nerve) enters the tympanic cavity in the hypotympanum, courses across the promontory, and exits just medial to the cochleariformis process. It then enters the middle fossa as the lesser superficial petrosal nerve and exits through a fissure or foramen of its own, terminating in the otic ganglion.

The Inner Ear

The inner ear consists of three semicircular canals, the vestibule, and the cochlea (Fig. 2–5). The bone or labyrinth of the inner ear is compact and very dense. The labyrinth is suspended in a latticework of air cells within the apex of the temporal bone. Inside this bony structure is a membranous labyrinth.

Semicircular Canals

Because this discussion is primarily concerned with the auditory system, the vestibular apparatus will not be discussed in detail There are three

Figure 2–5.   The inner ear consists of the three semicircular canals, the vestibule, and the cochlea.

semicircular canals: the horizontal or lateral, the posterior, and the superior. These canals open into the vestibule, the superior and posterior canals having a common crus. Thus, there are three semicircular canals with five openings into the vestibule. Each canal contains a corresponding membranous counterpart. There is an ampulated or swollen end of each canal containing the neuroepithelium of the peripheral vestibular system.

Vestibule

The vestibule is the central part of the osseous labyrinth lying between the semicircular canals and the cochlea. Its medial wall has two depressions, the recessus ellipticus, which holds the membranous utricle, and the recessus sphericus, in which the saccule rests. Running parallel to the common crus is the opening for the vestibular aqueduct. The medial wall is perforated, allowing the fibers of the vestibular nerve to enter the utricle, the saccule, and the superior and horizontal ampulae.

Cochlea

The cochlea is the peripheral center for hearing and is an extremely complicated structure. Its bony contours resemble a common snail shell, as its coil makes approximatley two and two-thirds turns. Measuring about 5 mm from base to apex and 9 mm across its base, the cochlea contains a conical-shaped central axis known as the modiolus, from which projects a delicate ledge of bone—the osseous spiral lamina. Extending from the spiral lamina is the basilar membrane separating the cochlea into two chambers that communicate with each other at the apex of the modiolus by a small opening—the helicotrema.

The modiolus is the central conical core of the cochlea, wide at the base and narrow at the apex. The bony canal of the cochlea is about 30 mm in length and approximately 3 mm in diameter and communicates through three openings to other structures: The round window (fenestra rotundum) is closed by the round window membrane, the second opening connects the cochlea to the vestibule, and the cochlear aqueduct communicates with the subarachnoid space. The latter structure transmits cerebrospinal fluid from the subarachnoid space into the scala tympani of the cochlea.

The cochlea is divided into three separate chambers by the osseous lamina, the basilar membrane, and Reissner's membrane (Fig. 2–6). The chambers are the scala media (cochlear duct), the scala vestibuli, and the scala tympani. The scala media is formed by the basilar and Reissner's membranes and contains the organ of Corti, which sits on the inner part of the basilar membrane. The organ of Corti consists of epithelial elements forming two rows of rod-like bodies known as the inner and outer rods or pillars of Corti. The bases of the pillars are supported on the

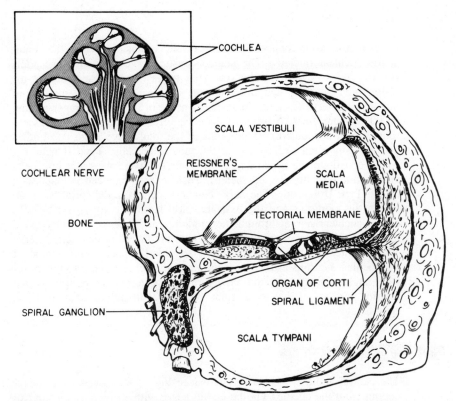

Figure 2–6. The cochlea is divided into three separate chambers by the osseous lamina, the basilar membrane, and Reissner's membrane.

basilar membrane, and the tops incline toward each other to form an arch or tunnel of Corti. The inner row of rods contain the inner hair cells (single), whereas the outer side of the rods support three or four rows of similar cells, termed the supporting cells of Dieters and Hensen. The free ends of the outer hair cells are embedded in the tectorial membrane. The inner hair cells number about 3500 and the outer hair cells number about 12,000.

Along the outer aspect of the scala media lies the stria vascularis, a vascular meshwork of arteries, which is thought to produce endolymph, the clear fluid found throughout the membranous labyrinth. The scala vestibuli and tympani, bony vestibule, and bony semicircular canals contain a clear fluid, perilymph, which is thought to arise from the cerebrospinal fluid through the cochlear aqueduct. Perilymph and endolymph are similar in nature, but endolymph is high in potassium ion concentration and perilymph is high in sodium ion concentration.

The Auditory Nerve

First order neurons connect the cochlea to the brainstem, where they enter at the cochlear nucleus. The staticoacoustic nerve (cranial nerve VIII) consists of two divisions: the vestibular nerve (superior and inferior divisions and Scarpa's ganglion) and the cochlear nerve. The number of myelinating nerve fibers in the cochlear nerve of humans averages around 35,000. There are two types of cochlear afferent neurons. Type I neurons, which account for 95 per cent of the total, have large cell bodies and are connected exclusively to the inner hair cells. Type II neurons, which constitute the remaining 5 per cent, innervate the outer hair cells and do not have myelinated sheaths. Each interval hair cell is innervated by ten Type II neurons. The nerve cells are located in the spiral ganglion within the modiolus and the osseous spiral lamina. Axons pass by way of the cochlear nerve through the modiolus and internal auditory canal and across the cerebellopontine angle with the facial nerve (cranial nerve VII) to enter the brainstem. There is an orderly spatial arrangement of the cochlear neurons as they pass through the cochlear nerve to the brainstem nuclei. Fibers from the basal turn are located in the peripheral and inferior portions of the nerve trunk, and apical fibers are situated in the central region.

Central Auditory Pathways

The central auditory nervous system (see Fig. 2–7) receives the neural coding from the cochlea via the eighth nerve with an increasing order of complexity. At least in such animals as the monkey, the cochlear nucleus is estimated to have 88,000 cells while the cortex has 10,000,000, with an increase at each level above the cochlear nucleus.[4] In addition to the forwarding of auditory signals, the system also incorporates input and output intersensory connections as well as connections to motor systems.

Cochlear Nucleus

The cochlear nucleus is on the lateral edge of the hindbrain. Its three major subdivisions are the anterior ventral cochlear nucleus, the posterior ventral nucleus, and the dorsal cochlear nucleus. All eighth-nerve fibers reach two of these three areas. All proceed to the anterior ventral nucleus and simultaneously to one of the other divisions. As in the cochlea, the arrangement and distribution of fibers crossing these three areas is frequency oriented. However, because of the much more complicated array of response units, significant temporal manipulation apparently begins even at this relatively low level.

Second order fibers leave the cochlear nucleus in three groups: the dorsal, the intermediate, and the ventral striae. The ventral group (the trapezoid body) sends medial and ventral projections terminating in the

Figure 2–7. The distal projections from the inferior colliculus are primarily to the medial geniculate body and thence to the auditory cortex in the temporal lobe of the brain.

lateral superior olive, the medial superior olive, and the medial nucleus of the trapezoid body. At this point, these fibers cross to the contralateral medial superior olive and trapezoid body. Ipsilateral fibers go to the lateral superior olive. The intermediate acoustic stria enters the dorsal portion of the superior olivary complex, then crosses to the contralateral side to the lateral lemniscus, some fibers ascending to the inferior colliculus. The dorsal acoustic stria bypasses the superior olivary complex and synapses in the contralateral dorsal nuclei of the lateral lemniscus and the inferior colliculus.

Superior Olivary Complex

The superior olivary complex is the earliest junction of signals from both cochleae. This junction consists of the lateral and medial superior olive, the medial nucleus of the superior olive, and the lateral lemniscus. The medial superior olive receives fibers from both cochleae but more directly from the ipsilateral side so that it has primitive timing functions. The lateral superior olive receives only ipsilateral cochlear fibers directly and delayed messages from the contralateral side by way of the medial trapezoid body. These pathways appear most useful in detecting amplitude (or intensity) differences to the two ears on simultaneous presentation.

The response is more likely to be activated by ipsilateral stimulation and depressed by contralateral stimulation.

At least part of the function of the superior olivary complex is to provide primitive information to the brain for purposes of localization. The acoustic stapedial reflex and the aural–palpebral reflex appear to mediate at this level.

Lateral Lemniscus

The lateral lemniscus is the next major synapse. It is located on the lateral edge of the pons. Little of its auditory input is binaural and consists of the dorsal, intermediate, and ventral nuclei of the lateral lemniscus and forwards information to the midbrain. The response units are most sensitive to contralateral stimulation. Its function may be that of a dumb relay, although there is little known about this level of transmission in the brainstem for auditory processing.

Inferior Colliculus

Information, however altered at the superior olivary complex or lateral lemniscus, is received in the auditory midbrain at the inferior colliculus. All ascending auditory fibers synapse here. Information is received from both ears coming in part directly as low as the contralateral cochlear nucleus. The afferent auditory fibers enter the ventrolateral portion of the central nucleus of the inferior colliculus. The majority of cochlear nucleus fibers have crossed to the contralateral dorsal cochlear nucleus and ascended to the inferior colliculus. Some smaller portion of fibers come from the ipsilateral medial and lateral superior olive, again with tonotopic frequency organization.

Medial Geniculate Body

The auditory portion of the thalamus, the medial geniculate body, receives input from the inferior colliculus and from the cortex. There is only same-side interaction at this level. Again, tonotopic information is forwarded to the primary auditory cortex but without any recoding.

Auditory Cortex

The auditory areas of the cerebral cortex are in the Sylvian fissure at the superior temporal gyrus in the neighboring cortex and in the parietal operculum. This central processing area receives information from the ascending nuclei in tonotopic arrangement with surrounding areas providing connection to other sensory input systems and response mode. This area is a complex integration system for both reflex and intellective responses. Its complexity exceeds the present discussion, but it is concerned with observing signal intensity, frequency characteristics, and location and comparing these to what is already known about the outside world. Observations of its function and dysfunction are beyond analysis with ABR and are therefore omitted from further discussion.

Efferent Pathways

Although the efferent pathways will receive increasing attention and have undoubted significance in evaluating auditory response, they are poorly understood at this point. Their influence on the ABR, which may be considerable, is not documented, and to describe them for clinical application would be unrealistic.

PHYSIOLOGY OF THE AUDITORY SYSTEM

The function of the auditory system is dependent on three factors: (1) the structural composition of the outer, middle, and inner ear; (2) the production of electrical impulses originating in the cochlea; and (3) the transmission of these impulses through the cochlear nerve and the central neural pathways.

The Mechanism of Hearing

The auricle is of little auditory significance in the human. Its location on either side of the head provides an acoustic baffle between the two ears in order to assure that the direction of sound can be detected. In humans the whole head is used to scan for sound as opposed to the individual scanning ability of the auricle in lower animal forms. Sound is created by vibrations of air particles, which are collected by the auricle and external canal and are then transmitted to the tympanic membrane. The chief function of the middle ear is to provide an impedance match between the air of the external auditory canal and the fluid of the cochlea, thereby efficiently delivering acoustic energy to the organ of Corti.

The external auditory canal has a resonant frequency of 4000 Hertz (Hz), which accounts for an increase of sensitivity of about 10 dB at this frequency. The middle ear has a resonant frequency of approximately 1700 Hz. Therefore, combined with the external canal, the overall acoustic frequency response of the ear is 800 to 6000 Hz.

The vibrating air particles set the tympanic membrane into motion, which, in turn, drives the ossicular chain. The large surface area of the tympanic membrane—80 mm^2—compared to the small area of the stapes footplate—3 mm^2—creates a hydraulic effect in a 20:1 ratio, which allows the weak air vibrations to set the perilymph of the vestibule into motion.

As the stapes moves into the vestibule, a traveling wave is set up in the basilar membrane moving toward the scala tympani. The round window membrane bulges outward to compensate for the inward motion of the stapes, since the fluid cannot be compressed. When the movement is slow, some fluid also flows through the helicotrema. The basilar membrane is narrow at the base and wide at the apex, so that high frequencies are detected in the base and low frequencies in the apex. Thus, the cochlea is a mechanical frequency analyzer. As the basilar membrane bulges in response to vibrations of the stapes footplate, the hair cells of the organ of Corti are bent by the movement of the tectoral membrane. Bending of the hair cells releases energy in the form of bioelectric potentials, which are responsible for excitation of the auditory nerve fibers. The electrical activity is then transmitted by the cochlear nerve to the central pathways and by way of the brainstem to the auditory cortex, where integration takes place.

Electrical Responses of the Cochlea

The electrical activity of the central nervous system can be detected on the body surface and recorded, thus making possible the science of electrocardiography (ECG) and electroencephalography (EEG). Similarly, the electrical impulses generated by the cochlea and central auditory pathways can be detected and recorded, making electrocochleography (ECochG) and auditory brainstem response audiometry possible.

Action Potentials

If the electrical activity of the cochlea is synchronized into definite groups or volleys, as in response to clicks or successive sound waves of a low-frequency tone, the corresponding action potentials can be recorded by placing an electrode on the round window and one on the neck. Action potentials are recorded as the impulses pass through the modiolus just before they enter the internal auditory canal. Action potentials demonstrate an all-or-none "spike" response common to nerve fibers having a definite threshold followed by a refractory period.

Intracellular Potentials

With microelectrodes it is possible to measure the electric potential within a single cell. The intracellular potentials of the hair cells, nerve fibers, and supporting cells of the cochlea are negative and vary in strength from -80 to -20 millivolts (mv).

Endocochlear Potential

The endolymph in the scala media has a positive ($+80$ mv) electric potential relative to the perilymph in the scalae tympani and vestibuli as well as to the perilymph in the spiral ligament and extracochlear tissues. The so-called endocochlear potential is dependent on an adequate supply of oxygen and falls rapidly in the anoxic experimental animal. The endocochlear potential is modified with displacement of the structures within the cochlea. As the basilar membrane moves toward the scala tympani and the stapes are driven into the oval window, there is a 5- to 10-mv increase in the positive potential. Outward movement of the stapes produces a reduction in the potential. Changes in the endocochlear potential are related to displacement rather than velocity and are sustained as long as the displacement occurs.

The source of the endocochlear potential is the stria vascularis. The changes in the potential that occur with displacement are generated in the organ of Corti (hair cells), but this organ is not responsible for the resting positive potential.

Cochlear Microphonic and Summating Potentials

Acoustic stimulation by the bending of cochlear hair cells produces a cochlear microphonic (CM) and two summating potentials (SP), both positive and negative. The CM is directly proportional to the displacement of the cochlear partition and therefore reproduces the waveform of the acoustic stimulus. The summating potentials reproduce the form of an envelope of the original acoustic signal. Both the CM and SP are linear and are related to the intensity of the acoustic stimulus; they do not exhibit a "threshold" like that of all-or-none action potentials. There is no evidence to suggest an all-or-none response in the hair cells or of a refractory period; therefore the CM and the SP demonstrate little or no fatigue or adaptation.

The CM is dependent on oxygen, as is the endocochlear potential, but it is affected by certain injuries that leave the endocochlear potential intact.

The SP is observed on the oscilloscope as a displacement of the baseline record on which the CM is superimposed. With toxic injury to the cochlea (anoxia, and so forth), the CM decreases and the negative SP increases. Likewise, a decrease in the positive potential is accompanied by an increase in the negative potential. The positive and negative potentials are thought to originate in the inner hair cell system, whereas the CM and the positive SP probably arise in the external hair cells.

The full sequence of changes depends on the state of the cochlea, the position of the electrodes, and the frequency of the tone burst employed to produce the responses.

Volleys and Latencies

When the auditory nerve is stimulated with a single click, a sharp, well-synchronized volley of action potentials is produced. The initial response is referred to as N_1. Apparently N_1 and N_2 result from repetitive firing of some, but not all, of the fibers owing to the refractory period of nerve fibers (Fig. 2–8).

The successive sound waves of a steady tone between 2000 and

Figure 2–8. When the auditory nerve is stimulated with a single click, a sharp, well-synchronized volley of action potentials is produced. The initial response is referred to as N_1. Apparently N_1 and N_2 result from repetitive firing of some, but not all, of the fibers owing to the refractory period of nerve fibers.

4000 Hz give rise to similar, but smaller, volleys of action potentials that clearly reproduce the frequence of the tone, although no one fiber responds to every sound wave. At 1000 Hz or below, N_1 is produced in the basal turn of the cochlea, in which the partition moves almost in phase as a unit. Different latencies of response account for less and less perfect synchronization of the impulses as frequency increases. Above 4000 Hz there is no synchronization either visible on the oscilloscope or audible. By using a high-frequency tone burst there is a well-synchronized N_1 and N_2 and sometimes N_3. The latency of N_1 shortens from 2 milliseconds (msec) near threshold to 1 msec as intensity increases. Latency is related to rise-time, intensity, and frequency of the acoustic signal.

Latency of action potentials is a reflection of the conduction time within the nonmyelinated dendritic branches of the organ of Corti. As the volley passes through the modiolus it is recorded and measured from the beginning of the CM to the bottom of the action potential spike. There is no latency between the mechanical movement of the cochlear partition and the CM.

Below 3000 Hz, each sound wave acts more like an individual stimulus. Excitation occurs as the scalae media and vestibuli become more negative relative to the scala tympani, namely with outward movement of the stapes.

Single Fiber Activity

The single nerve fibers of the auditory system are 2.5 to 4.0 microns in diameter. If these fibers are probed with a microelectrode and the auditory system is stimulated with a brief tone burst, the resulting spike responses are similar to those from myelinated nerve fibers of similar size in other parts of the body. The auditory fibers give single or repetitive responses and will demonstrate either low or high thresholds. Most are selective with respect to frequency in that they demonstrate a sharp and stable cut-off frequency above which they fail to respond regardless of the intensity of the stimulation. Almost all fibers have cut-offs above 1000 Hz, but some have cut-offs as low as 100 Hz.

The phenomenon of adaptation is explained on the basis of a gradually diminishing rate of irregular discharges that continue after presenting a continuing tonal stimulation to the auditory nerve.

As the stimulus increases, N_1 increases along a sigmoid curve before reaching a plateau and once again rising much more rapidly. The tendency of single nerve fibers to group into high-threshold and low-threshold classes explains the nonlinear behavior of N_1 in the whole-nerve response.

Auditory Brainstem Activity

The fiber bundles ascending from the auditory nerve through the brainstem to the cortex are strictly organized tonotopically, as described in the preceding discussion of anatomy. Recoding of the sound pulse into intensity, temporal, and frequency cues is maintained and advanced both contralaterally and ipsilaterally until the information is deposited for cue integration and interpretation in the cortex. Of particular interest for the electrophysiologist are those fibers which are capable of synchronized discharge, a partial group of the cochlear network responding in the 2000 to 4000 Hz region. These fibers are able to fire with short rise time, recover rapidly, and can respond readily and consistently to a stimulus such as the rapid onset click. This capacity allows for a synchronous discharge efficient enough to be seen in an averaged auditory response.

Efferent Inhibitory Action

The efferent auditory pathway consists of fibers extending from the cortex to the cochlea. Stimulation of the olivocochlear tract (bundle of Rasmussen) in the medulla has an inhibitory effect on the action potential response to clicks. N_1 is reduced, but the CM is unaltered. The purpose of this efferent pathway is not understood.

PATHOPHYSIOLOGY OF THE AUDITORY SYSTEM

The normal transmission of sound waves through the middle ear, cochlea, and central pathways to the cerebral cortex presumes on a functioning auditory system. Pathologic changes can occur at any point in the mechanism, resulting in hearing loss or disruption of the orderly transfer of neural impulses through the brainstem pathways, which is referred to as dysynchrony.

Hearing Loss

There are three basic types of hearing loss: conductive, sensorineural, or a combination of the two, which is referred to as mixed loss.

Conductive Hearing Loss

Conductive losses are caused by blockage of sound vibrations in their transfer through the external auditory canal and middle ear. The simplest and one of the commonest forms of conductive hearing loss results from an accumulation of excessive cerumen in the external auditory canal (Fig. 2–9). The resulting hearing loss can reach 60 dB air conduction levels with impaction. Happily, this type of loss is easily reversible by removing the cerumen. A foreign body occluding the external canal is not an unusual finding. Children push pencils, erasers, beans, and all manner of small objects into their ears. Again, the loss is reversed by removing the foreign object.

Disease processes affecting the tympanic membrane and middle ear cavity are another cause of conductive hearing loss. A perforation of the eardrum, depending on its size and location, can be responsible for minimal to moderate conductive losses. The loss in this situation may depend on whether there is a phase difference between the oval and round windows. A perforation over the area of the round window will result in loss of protection to the phase difference and increase the severity of the loss (Fig. 2–10).

In chronic ear disease there may be a combination of pathologic processes accounting for the hearing loss. Not only is there a tympanic membrane perforation present but also associated with this may be a va-

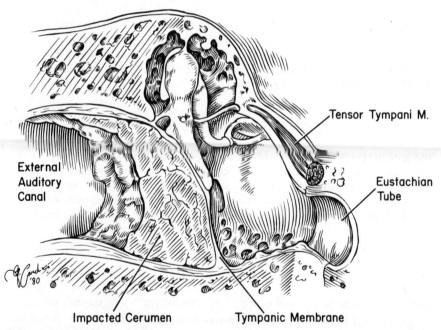

Figure 2–9. Conductive hearing losses are caused by blockage of sound vibrations in their transfer through the external auditory canal and middle ear. The simplest and one of the commonest forms of conductive hearing loss results from an accumulation of excessive cerumen in the external auditory canal.

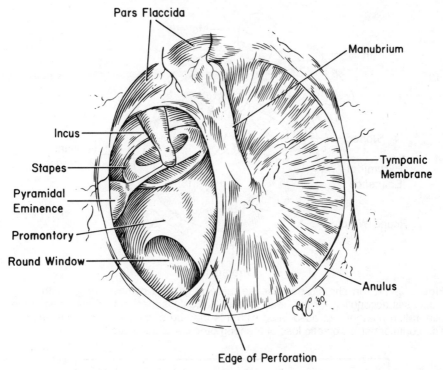

Pars Flaccida

Manubrium

Incus

Stapes

Pyramidal
Eminence

Promontory

Round Window

Tympanic
Membrane

Anulus

Edge of Perforation

Figure 2–10.   A perforation over the area of the round window will result in a loss of protection to the phase difference and increase the severity of the loss.

riety of ossicular defects. The commonest is necrotic loss of the long process of the incus (Fig. 2–11). A number of possible causes include loss of the superstructure of the stapes and of the handle of the malleus. Destruction of the ossicles may occur as a result of granulation tissue, repeated infections in the tympanic cavity, or cholesteatoma. Skin within the middle ear cleft or mastoid process causes a tremendous amount of destruction over a period of several years. Modern techniques of tympanoplasty, tympanoplasty with mastoidectomy, and methods of ossicular reconstruction make it possible in a high percentage of cases to repair the diseased middle ear and restore hearing.

In some instances the tympanic membrane itself appears normal, but a conductive hearing loss is evident. This situation usually indicates either fixation or discontinuity of the ossicular chain. Impedance audiometry is helpful in distinguishing between the two processes. Discontinuity may be the result of trauma or loss of the long process of the incus. Fixation may occur at the stapes owing to otosclerosis (Fig. 2–12) or a congenital absence of the anular ring of the footplate. Either problem can be corrected by stapedectomy. Occasionally the fixation involves the malleus head and body of the incus, whereas the stapes is freely mobile. This

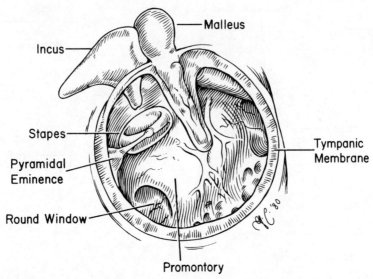

Figure 2–11. In chronic ear disease there may be a combination of pathologic processes accounting for the hearing loss. Not only is there a tympanic membrane perforation present, but associated with this may be a variety of ossicular defects. The commonest is necrotic loss of the long process of the incus.

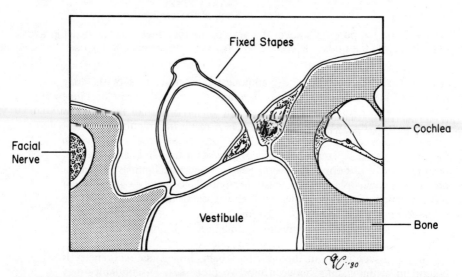

Figure 2–12. In some instances the tympanic membrane itself appears normal but a conductive hearing loss is evident. This situation usually indicates either fixation or discontinuity of the ossicular chain. Impedance audiometry is helpful in distinguishing between the two processes. Discontinuity may be the result of trauma or loss of the long process of the incus. Fixation may occur at the stapes owing to otosclerosis or a congenital absence of the anular ring of the footplate.

process is usually the result of tympanosclerotic plaques fixing the ossicles in the epitympanum. Hearing can be restored by removing the incus and the head of the malleus followed by reconstruction of the ossicular chain by sculpturing a prosthesis from the incus to fit between the handle of the malleus and the capitulum of the stapes.

Conductive hearing loss commonly occurs behind an intact tympanic membrane. In this situation serous otitis media resulting from eustachian tube malfunction produces a transudate of serous fluid from the mucous membrane lining the middle ear cleft (Fig. 2–13). As the tympanic cavity fills with fluid, the vibrating responses of the tympanic membranes are dampened, thereby creating a conductive loss. In some instances the fluid becomes viscid, accounting for the appellation "glue ear." Clear serous fluid can sometimes be removed from the middle ear simply by the Valsalva maneuver. The glue ear will not clear itself in this manner and requires myringotomy and forceful extraction of the material with a suction device.

Recently it has been popular to insert different types of ventilating tubes into the substance of the tympanic membrane to prevent the recurrence of the fluid. The middle ear cleft is ventilated through the plastic tube rather than the patient's eustachian tube. Once the fluid has been

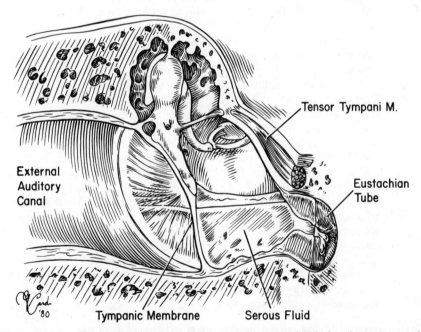

Figure 2–13. Conductive hearing loss commonly occurs behind an intact tympanic membrane. In this situation serous otitis media resulting from eustachian tube malfunction produces a transudate of serous fluid from the mucous membrane lining the middle ear cleft.

removed, and assuming the process does not repeat itself, hearing returns to normal levels.

In summary, conductive hearing losses are, by and large, amenable to some type of medical intervention.

Sensorineural Hearing Loss

As its name implies, sensorineural or sensory end-organ loss occurs when there is damage to or interference with the neural pathways of the auditory system. The conductive mechanism—external auditory canal, tympanic membrane, or ossicular chain—in these cases is usually normal. The cochlear partition is displaced by the movement of the stapes in a routine manner, but electrical impulses created in this manner do not reach the auditory cortex. The lesion may be limited to the hair cell system (sensory) or to the auditory nerve and central pathways (neural). For practical purposes, losses fitting into this category are not usually defined specifically as either sensory or neural in nature but are referred to simply as sensorineural. If the etiology of the loss is known, it is possible to state with some assurance which type it is. For example, since ototoxic antibiotics are known to destroy hair cells, a patient with a sensorineural loss who is on an antibiotic regimen probably has a sensory loss (Fig. 2–14). The individual with an acoustic tumor, however, would most likely have a neural loss (Fig. 2–15).

The widespread use of ECochG and ABR make it possible for clinicians to distinguish among the components of a sensorineural loss on a routine basis.

Sensorineural hearing loss may be caused by viral and bacterial infection, head injury or iatrogenic trauma, central nervous system disease such as acoustic tumors and intrinsic brainstem lesions, and as a result of congenital and hereditary defects. One of the most fascinating sensorineural hearing losses is that associated with Ménière's disease. The loss actually fluctuates from one day to another, sometimes by the hour, and will return to normal pure tone levels after an attack. Hydrops of the scala media (Fig. 2–16) may be the cause of the loss, in which case fluctuations can often be stabilized by salt restriction and the use of diuretics. Endolymphatic sac drainage surgery is offered to the individual who does not respond to medical management. If untreated, the process eventually destroys the contents of the cochlear partition, and in many cases the hearing loss progresses to become totally nonresponsive.

At the present state of the art, little if anything can be done to reverse the majority of sensorineural hearing losses, in contrast to conductive losses.

NEUROLOGIC DISORDERS INVOLVING THE BRAINSTEM

Theoretically, any disease process which is capable of interfering with neural transmission within the central pathways of the auditory system

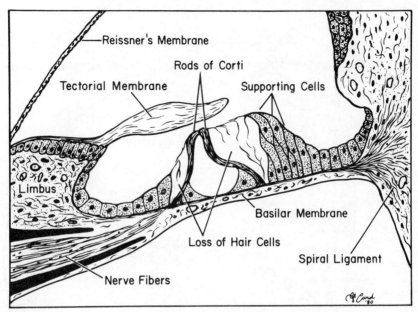

Figure 2–14. Since ototoxic antibiotics are known to destroy hair cells, a patient with a sensorineural loss who is on an antibiotic regimen probably has a sensory loss.

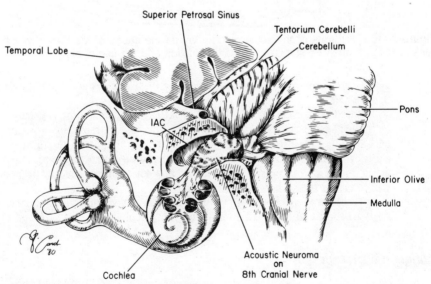

Figure 2–15. The individual with an accoustic tumor most likely would have a neural loss.

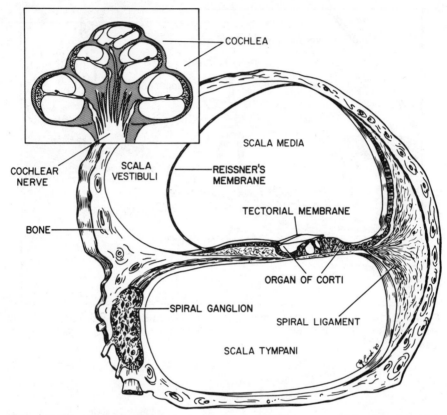

Figure 2–16. Hydrops of the scala media may be the cause of the loss in which fluctuations can often be stabilized by salt restriction and the use of diuretics.

might well produce a sensorineural hearing loss. The results of ABR may be affected.

Based on our current knowledge of ABR, we may assume that purely cortical disease, such as stroke, or cerebellar and extrapyramidal disorders such as Parkinson's disease will not alter the tracing. Although metabolic problems secondary to drug administration, even including anesthesia do not affect response latencies, we now know that severe intoxication will alter the ABR, as will hypothermia.[5]

The neurologic disorders most commonly associated with abnormal ABR tracings can be divided into two groups: congenital and acquired.

Congenital Disorders

There are primarily three congenital disorders which can affect the brainstem and thus the ABR in addition to other sensory and motor systems.

Prematurity is a common cause; there are so many potential sources of damage to the auditory system secondary to prematurity that abnormal ABR both neurologically and in terms of threshold is not unusual. This will be highlighted in Chapter 6. In addition, abnormal brainstem development (Moebius syndrome) and abnormal neuroectoderm development (anencephaly, hereditary leukodystrophy) will alter the ABR, among many other obvious signs of these developmental disorders.

Acquired Disorders

Acquired disorders may be divided into five categories: neoplasms, trauma, degenerative and demyelinating processes, infections, and vascular disorders.

Neoplasms

Intrinsic or extrinsic neoplasms of the brainstem will almost always alter the ABR. These would include acoustic neuromas, meningiomas, and primary cholesteatomas and other less common lesions of the cerebellopontine angle and internal auditory canal. Mass lesions can invade the eighth nerve or compress it or its blood supply, causing changes in neural transmission that often include reduced threshold sensitivity and speech discrimination ability. A large mass (more than four centimeters) can act as a lesion extrinsic to the brainstem and cause more central effects noted on contralateral test as well. A glomus jugulare tumor can infiltrate the cerebellopontine angle and act as an extrinsic lesion, resulting in retrocochlear test findings.

Intra-axial brainstem tumors include several groups of tissue types such as astrocytomas, glioblastomas, ependymomas, gliomas, and so on, with nomenclature reflecting the nature of the cell structures in the mass. Some of these lesions can be surgically removed in whole or part; some are sensitive to chemotherapy or radiation treatment resulting in cure or remission. Some are fatal. These lesions, which certainly do not selectively affect the auditory pathways, may yield a variety of abnormal patterns from normal peripheral sensitivity with abnormal ABR response to profound central signs. In like fashion the ABR may show any sort of configuration, from normal sequence, when the eigth nerve and brainstem are intact to no response or markedly bizarre pattern.

Trauma

An individual experiencing a head injury might well develop an epidural, subdural, or intracerebral hemorrhage with lower brainstem compression secondary to central nervous system shift. Fractures of the temporal bone with involvement of the cochlear nerve or middle ear ossicles might cause ABR alterations as well. Isolation of these effects of trauma must be undertaken before identification of neural impairment can be made. Recent studies in monitoring trauma patients have suggested that the ABR may be a prognostic factor in rating the patient's likelihood of recovery. These predictions are made on the basis of serial recordings initiated as soon as possible after the patient comes to evaluation.[6]

Degenerative and Demyelinating Processes

An example of a degenerative processs would be the adult form of leukodystrophy. The three most common demyelinating processes that will affect ABR are multiple sclerosis, Schilder's diffuse cerebral sclerosis, and hermorrhagic leukoencephalopathies. Generally patients with multiple sclerosis, the most common presentation, will have several seemingly unrelated complaints and describe periods of remission. Although loss of sensitivity is uncommon, alterations in ABR are more common—60% or more—according to Robinson and Rudge.[7] Sclerotic placques may occur throughout the brain and spinal cord. The ABR pattern can vary immensely, with only minimal indication of eighth nerve integrity to markedly bizarre sequences, at times apparently unstable even on immediate retest.

Infections

Infections are usually viral and would include anything that would involve white matter in the brainstem such as bulbar poliomyelitis or encephalitis. Another example is the sudden hearing loss caused in some cases by herpes zoster oticus. The effect may be both in the cochlea and the eighth nerve (as well as the facial and trigeminal nerves). The auditory tests, including ABR, will sometimes reflect the retrocochlear changes in some of these patients. Syphilis, a common source of cochlear changes, may more rarely affect the eighth nerve along with other sensory nerves and the brain. Resulting changes are unpredictable, although they are occasionally reflected in an abnormal ABR trace.

Vascular Disorders

Cerebrovascular disorders may or may not be transient. They include such disorders as atherosclerosis, arteriosclerosis (a by-product of hypertension), arteriovenous malformations, aneurysms, and intrinsic trauma or stroke. Diabetes mellitus, a chronic systemic disease, may cause vascular disorders resulting in both cochlear and eighth nerve changes.

It is not within the scope of this book to attempt a detailed list of neurologic disorders affecting ABR. One must be aware of the fact, however, that a prolonged or absent wave V is not pathognomonic of an acoustic tumor. The diagnosis of this lesion must be accomplished by means of posterior fossa myelogram or computerized axial tomography (CAT) scanning. Perhaps it is well to point out now, as the text will illustrate in later chapters, that ABR is not a test of anatomy; it is a test of function, normal and abnormal.

REFERENCES

1. Gray, H.: *Anatomy of the Human Body*. Philadelphia, Lea & Feibeger,
2. Schuknecht, H. F.: *Pathology of the Ear*. Cambridge, Harvard University Press, 1974.
3. Davis, H. F.: Principles of electric response audiometry. Ann Otol Rhinol Laryngol 85 (Suppl 28):1–96, 1976.
4. Chow, K. L. Numerical estimates of the auditory central nervous system of the rhesus monkey. J Comp Neurol 95:159–175, 1951.
5. Stockard, J. J., Stockard, J. G., and Sharbrough, F. W.: Nonpathological factors influencing brainstem auditory evoked potentials. Am J EEG Technol 18:177–209, 1978.
6. Hecox, K.: Personal communication, 1982.
7. Robinson, K., and Rudge, P.: Abnormalities of the auditory evoked potentials in patients with multiple sclerosis. Brain 100:19–40, 1977.

CHAPTER THREE

INSTRUMENTATION AND BASIC TECHNIQUE

INTRODUCTION

This chapter is organized to present an overview of the principles and the techniques for auditory brainstem response audiometry as a background for practical applications and is not intended to be a comprehensive explanation of computer analysis procedures. There follows a review of instrumentation, techniques, calibration procedures, and troubleshooting suggestions. Even clinicians concerned primarily with test interpretation rather than test technique should be aware of the following principles.

BIOLOGICAL AVERAGING

Biological averaging allows extraction of a small target signal from random noise. A measurable auditory evoked potential requires synchronous discharge from the cochlea. Such a response can be elicited by a carefully selected stimulus such as a click. Latency of the response to the click depends on sound intensity and the sensitivity of the system being tested.

Principles of Averaging

Signal averaging involves analysis of a number of response samples, amplifying the target response while eliminating other activity or "noise." The background noise at the scalp is the ongoing electroencephalic activity, a relatively large amount of noise in comparison to the small voltage of the ABR. The electroencephalic activity produces a random signal with no particular pattern or cycle; that is, it is not time-locked to the onset of the stimulus. When an appropriate acoustic signal is intense enough to evoke an action potential, a small direct current potential is triggered and creates a wave of positive and negative variations relative to the electroencephelogram (EEG) potentials as the sound-generated impulse completes each neuronal transfer from the cochlea through the auditory nerve and brainstem. Although these events are stable without averaging, these minute electrical changes will be unobservable at the vertex electrode because of the comparatively large voltage of the EEG. The background electrical activity is generally on the order of 10 microvolts (μv) at the scalp.[1] In contrast, the auditory brainstem responses are on the order of 0.01 to 1 μv.[2] With such a large difference between the noise and the target response signal, observation of a single auditory response is not feasible. The problem, then, is to eliminate "noise" while enhancing the auditory responses. The solution is averaging.

Changes in potential are recorded from the onset of each stimulation to the end of the desired time interval. The averager breaks down this time assignment into "storage bins." In each bin or division the averager stores the relative electric potential present at that poststimulus time until the run or "epoch" is completed. The averager starts sampling at the instant the click drives the earphone and stops at a set interval after stimulation (for auditory brainstem responses, generally 10 milliseconds [msec] after stimulation). This time period allows evaluation of the brainstem responses in normal adults but must be expanded for some patient responses. Let us assume that the measuring time, called the "gate" or epoch, is 10 msec. At 0 msec the time triggers the stimulus to the cochlea and the computer starts checking each stack or resolution point for storage of the EEG data over the 10-msec period and repeats the procedure until the designated number of sweeps is completed. At the onset of the signal, the sweep begins and stores the data of each time division in a series of rows or columns and repeats this procedure several times. These columns, whose number is determined by computer design, can build above or fall below the relative zero line at each part of a millisecond that the electrical activity is measured. If there is virtually no relative potential at 0.10 msec, that block will be a relatively small contribution to the column. Conversely, continuing with this example, at 5.50 msec a large positive block would be stacked, representing a significant voltage increase, followed at 5.6 msec with a large relative negative voltage. Having stored information for 10 msec the averager will start the collection again at zero, adding voltages in the second run to the columns and so on until the predetermined number of sweeps is reached. Then the averager analyzes the data and provides the arithmetic mean of the data input. If the system being measured is normal, the response will appear as five to seven "bumps," generally designated as the Jewett[3] sequence. This straight-line average with no signal and the resulting change with auditory response are shown in Figures 3–1 and 3–2.

Because the gate is synchronized only to the acoustic signal, random electrical noise such as the ongoing cortical activity, movement, myogenic response, and so on will be averaged to zero. Current computer technique is such that time-locked responses add in a linear fashion, whereas random responses add as the square root of the number of stimulations. That is, repeating the sweet 100 times will result in a 10:1 signal-to-noise improvement. Thus, at very large samples, most computer systems can

Figure 3–1. Example of average of random activity (no sound). Line represents averaged activity to ±0.5 volts for 1024 samples at eight samples per second, with the subject asleep.

add only a small increase in the signal-to-noise ratio, and for some equipment the desired response actually becomes blunted in the additional averaging.

Averagers store the information digitally. In most clinically designed systems at present the signals are coded by analogue and are converted to digital code in the A-to-D converter, so that the voltages are stored as two-digit numbers. Conversion is made for each point of evaluation during the present time for every run and is averaged at the conclusion. To obtain sufficient analysis, 12-bit amplitude resolution is considered sufficient, and the averager should provide time base 256 words of a 24-bit length.

In summary, the purpose of averaging is simply to enhance the target response while minimizing background noise. Ability to detect the brainstem auditory responses is also dependent on proper instrumentation and test technique. Figure 3-3 outlines some of the sections that will be discussed below.

INSTRUMENTATION

Preamplifier

The preamplifier applies the principle of common mode rejection (CMR) for further enhancement of the signal. In a differential amplifier, voltages

Figure 3–2. Same conditions as in Figure 3–1, except that the average is time-locked to an acoustical stimulus, a click (0.1 msec at 50 dB above threshold for the stimulus). These baseline changes in the average represent the (del) auditory brainstem responses known as the Jewett sequence.

Figure 3–3. Block diagram for recording auditory evoked potentials.

observed at the active electrode are subtracted from those at the reference
or indifferent electrode by reversing its polarity. The result is cancellation
of all voltage activity common to both electrodes. Through this CMR the
target signal becomes the primary electric input for amplification and data
storage. CMR allows cancellation of such artifacts as 60-cycle interference or random internal responses. The ability of the equipment to provide such a function is expressed as the "CMR ratio," the ratio of the
two outputs when some specified signal is applied. A high rejection rate
is desirable.

Because the preamplifier has the task of boosting the signal on the
order of 10^6, its own internal noise characteristics must be known. The
internal noise level is determined by measuring noise present when the
preamplifier leads are shorted. Because it is impossible to eliminate
preamplifier noise completely, the best compromise is a preamplifier that
is specified to have low internal noise. As high input impedance is also
desirable, there is a certain amount of trade-off involved. Generally 10
μv peak-to-peak internal noise with 50 megohms input impedance is acceptable.

In addition to providing CMR and a relatively quiet boost of the target signal, the preamplifier improves the auditory response through filtering. Most amplifiers are designed with broad frequency response, normally 1 Hertz (Hz) to 10 kilohertz (kHz). If the system's frequency response is altered to filter out undesired noise in low- and high-frequency ranges containing little or no auditory response, the resulting average will be easier to analyze. Clinical studies[4-6] suggests 3 kHz (3 decibels [dB] down) as the high cutoff, but there is less agreement regarding a low pass setting. Coats and Martin[4] suggest 50 Hz, Jerger and colleagues[5] 300 Hz, and Selters and Brackmann[6] 30 Hz. this variation depends in part on other response characteristics of the equipment in use and in part on the information desired in the average. In our experience the auditory brainstem responses are enhanced with 50 or 100 Hz low pass.

Finally, because the preamplifier must also provide patient protection to minimize shock hazard, clinical units are designed to isolate the patient from the instrument power.

Digital Section

The filtered amplified analogue signal is fed from the preamplifier to the digital section of the averager, where it is stored in the memory. In the A-to-D converter it is possible to provide artifact rejection, so that maximum use of the memory will be available to retain relevant signals instead of averaging noise. Artifact rejection simply involves discarding any sweeps with more than a specified number of off-scale points. Some clinical units use a preset, often at 5 percent. Others vary the acceptable percentage of off-scale points. In difficult situations it may be possible to obtain a recognizable Jewett series even though some off-scale data are allowed into the averager. One of our subjects, a patient with chronic spasms of the neck muscles, provided noisy but identifiable, repeatable responses with only artifact rejection eliminated from the system. With artifact rejection at 5 percent, too few acceptable responses were obtained after 5 minutes of attempts at 10 pulses per second (pps) to complete a sample of 512 responses. However, if no response can be observed under these conditions, it is not possible to make any interpretation of the results. Artifact rejection is an important asset in eliminating test artifact noise, though flexibility is desirable.

The digital section stores the voltages as a series of binary numbers called "bits," which represent each sample point and stores them as "words." To provide sufficient amplitude resolution for signal conversion, 12 bits are desirable. The averager takes these digitized data into the memory, where a true arithmetic average is maintained. Sufficient memory is provided by a unit with 24 bits with a minimum of 256 A-to-D conversion points. Some clinical units also provide for splitting the memory so that more than one run can be retained and superimposed for verification of retest of the response. In the averager there is a final conversion of the stored digital information to analogue form for display on an oscilloscope.

Recorders

There are several methods for permanent recording of the response. They can be retained in digital form on computer tape. In most clinical settings, however, it is more practical to record the oscilloscope signal with a strip chart recorder or X-Y plotter. Some clinicians have employed a camera—a slow process but useful in special situations such as the operating room. These responses can also be stored by the computer on retrievable storage such as diskettes for transfer to hard copy.

Stimulus Section

Another major phase of instrumentation is the stimulus section. For acquisition of clinically useful responses, the stimulus must be capable of provoking synchronous discharge of a large number of fibers. A signal producing such a large action potential must have a rapid rise time. Several types of signals are capable of producing enough response synchrony to yield a visible Jewett sequence. The pure tone stimulus produced by standard clinical audiometers has such a slow rise time that cochlear response is too desynchronized to be visible in the ongoing activity. A click, however, readily produced with a fast rise time (1 msec or less),[1] can elicit a response easily averaged out of the ongoing EEG. Synchrony is achieved both by onset characteristics and by frequency components. The stimulus must contain sufficient high-frequency to initiate discharge from the basal turn of the cochlea. Responses from the lower-frequency ranges of the medial and apical regions of the cochlea are less reliable or too desynchronous to be extracted directly from the other neuroelectric potentials.

Currently there are several types of stimuli that will provide good ABR data:

1. *The broad band click or square wave*. This stimulus meets the need for fast rise time and since it has a broad frequency range of energy, it will stimulate the high-frequency region important for a recordable brainstem response. Its duration must be as brief as possible, well under 1 msec, for use in averaged response audiometry. Although its electrical waveform is that of a rectangular pulse, the acoustic response will have peaks reflecting the transducer characteristics.

2. *Filtered clicks*. These stimuli are also easily produced and are more specific in stimulation. They are generated by ringing a third-octave bandpass filter with a raw click or single sine wave. Click duration is a function of the filter frequency. The advantage of filtering is the produc-

tion of more selective frequency stimulation, which is important in threshold ABR.

3. *Tone pips.* These signals are another alternative with adequate rise time characteristics and frequency specificity. The signal is a pure tone gated to control rise time and plateau for a given frequency, so that it produces a narrow peak at the indicated frequency as measured at the transducer. Davis[1] described use of this stimulus down to 1000 Hz to predict audiometric response curve.

4. *Single cycle pip.* This variant is formed by gating the tone from peak to peak to produce rapid rise time with tone-specific character. This signal is technically more difficult to produce but is less affected by transducer characteristics.

5. *Logon.* The Gaussian logon is a pure tone that is amplitude-modulated across a Gaussian distribution curve and is the best compromise between ideal frequency and rapid rise time according to Davis.[1] The logon is produced as a brief pip gated on and off over the distribution curve, so that it is much like a filtered click, and acoustically it presents a broad peak at the pip frequency.

The stimulus generator should also provide control of signal polarity. In difficult recording sites, the polarity of the signal can be alternated to obtain cancellation of artifact and cochlear microphonic (CM). Because there are special situations in which observation of the microphonic is desirable, the stimulus section should provide the capability of alternating polarity and providing a choice of compression or rarefaction phases. It should be noted that response interpretation will be significantly affected by this variable, and latency data will vary depending on choice of polarity.

Since stimulus characteristics are variable and are not standardized for ABR, reports of such criteria as normal range of latency and other response data must be understood as peculiar to that laboratory and not directly transferable to another set of circumstances. That is, latency and amplitude data cannot be compared from one clinic to another without concession to differences in instrumentation and procedure. Table 3–1 gives some idea of the range variability of stimuli employed by different investigators. The signal also provides a means for controlling stimulus duration. A 100 microsecond (μsec) click is a frequently recommended duration because it provides enough energy over time for threshold integration at relatively soft sensation levels, whereas shorter bursts compromise the maximum hearing loss which can be assessed by about 13 dB, according to Beattie and Boyd.[7] Longer signals require an adjustment in normative latency data. The same is true for tone pips.

The stimulus section must also provide a means of intensity control. The intensity is variably specified in terms of reference to a normal jury of hearers (dB nHL) or in terms of peak equivalent sound pressure level (peSPL) with 0.0002 microbar reference. The upper limit of available power is determined in part by the nature of the stimulus and the trans-

TABLE 3–1. Stimulus Variations in Several ABR Laboratories

Source	Stimulus
Selters and Brackmann[6]	160 microsec DC pulse applied 20 pps to earphones
Mokotoff, Schulmann-Galambos, Galambos[8]	0.1 msec square wave
Stockard and Rossiter[9]	Acoustic transients 0.1 msec
Starr and Hamilton[10]	"Clicks"
Davis[1]	Brief (0.2 msec or less) click at 1.2 and 4 Hz tone pips
Coats and Martin[4]	0.02 msec square wave pulse
Clemis and McGee[11]	Tone pip 1 msec rise and decay with total duration 2 msec (no plateau)
Glasscock et al.[12]	0.1 msec click (see Fig. 3–4).

ducer, but should be on the order of 130 dB peSPL and should allow variation downward to 0 dB peSPL to allow for threshold testing and other intensity variation procedures. (Techniques for determining output are suggested under the section on calibration.)

The stimulus section should include a timer to activate the averager simultaneously with the stimulus onset. It should allow variation in repetition rate from sufficiently slow to allow adequate recovery—generally under 20 pulses per second—to rapid for both site-of-lesion and threshold procedures. Note that because the stimuli are below critical duration, threshold is achieved at greater intensity than for a stimulus of standard duration matched in frequency. Direct inferences of threshold based on peSPL must take this difference into account. The basis for selecting repetition rate is presented later in this chapter.

Finally, the stimulus section includes the transducer. The stimulus can drive a free-field speaker, although this complicates monitoring intensity of signal at the eardrum, or it can be presented through an earphone. Because the response characteristics of the standard TDH 49 earphone can affect the high-frequency character of the stimulus, other earspeakers are sometimes preferred. For special test problems, a bone conduction transducer is a helpful addition. (See Chapter 4.)

Electrodes

A final consideration in instrumentation is the link of the patient to the preamplifier. The response generated by the appropriately prescribed stimulus must be detected for delivery to the preamplifier. The sensors, scalp electrodes, pick up the preliminary scalp potentials including EEG noise, artifact and auditory potential. Most commonly, gold or silver–silver chloride discs acting as volume conductors applied with reduced skin resistance (generally under 5000 ohms) will provide adequate signal input. The electrodes sense response of the various auditory generators, acting as dipoles, depending on their proximity and relative signal strength. If the dipole is oriented toward the electrode, the measured discharge will appear greater. That is, if the active electrode is at the vertex in parallel with the electric potential changes, the response will have the greatest volume. As opposed to some electroencephalographic procedures, the monopolar technique for recording auditory response results in less distortion than bipolar measures.[13]

In summary, instrumentation requires appropriate stimuli to elicit a detectable response at the surface electrodes. This signal is boosted and refined in the preamplifier, is converted to numerical data for averaging, and is stored in the digital section with final reproduction to visual representation on the oscilloscope.

TECHNIQUE

Introduction

Brainstem audiometric technique varies, depending on the purpose of the procedure—either site of lesion assessment or threshold determination. This section will describe some of the techniques of response acquisition and analysis.

Electrodes

There are several successful techniques for application and placement of electrodes to eliminate the problems of noise and poor retest. It is important to place the active electrode in the vicinity of C_z, the vertex. It can be located by intersecting lines joining nasion to inion and the preauricular points. The amplitude of the responses and polarity will vary depending on the relative position of the active electrode. For best analysis of the Jewett sequence the electrode should approximate C_z, although a slight variation has a limited effect. There are advocates of forehead placement for the active site to avoid problems of placing the electrode in hair, but this procedure alters responses at the level of waves IV and V. Since wave V in a normal subject has large amplitude, it will be visible with the active electrode at the forehead. However, in a patient with an abnormally decreased response amplitude, the response may appear to be absent or less repeatable with such an angled placement. Figure 3–4 compares forehead and vertex responses from a patient diagnosed as having multiple sclerosis and demonstrates this distortion.

Although the active electrode needs to be seated at the vertex for maximum amplitude of wave V, successful placement of the reference electrode varies. Sites include the ipsilateral mastoid, earlobe (front or back), and neck. None is truly indifferent, though the earlobe tends to have the least active participation. In our experience, neck placement has

Figure 3–4. Example of varying active electrode placement on a patient with abnormal response, active at forehead in top three traces, at C^Z on lower three traces. Reference to ipsilateral mastoid, at 60 dB above patient threshold for click, 8 pps.

proved a problem because of neuromuscular potentials. In general, the ipsilateral site is the reference, and the contralateral ear serves as the ground. Some investigators add a fourth electrode as a ground, placed equidistant between right and left references and roughly perpendicular to the line of travel of the auditory potential. The nasion is a common choice for the site; however, in our experience the addition of the fourth electrode has not improved clinical interpretation or response reliability over pairing with the opposite site in single-channel recordings. Two-channel recordings, however, will call for interplay of electrode array to heighten or minimize certain segments of the recording. For example, with "ground" at the nasion and active at the vertex, a two-channel recording might simultaneously gather data from the ipsilateral ear (side of sound stimulation) to the vertex and from the contralateral ear to the vertex. Because the off-side record helps to separate wave IV from V, it can aid in the process of locating the point to identify as wave V. Other electrode arrays, for example from contralateral to ipsilateral ear, can sometimes aid in the identification of wave I. Morgan and associates[14] found that multichannel recording heightened confidence in wave identification and provided improved definition of waves IV and V.

To obtain adequate recordings from any of these far-field sites, electrodes must be applied meticulously. Sufficient reduction in skin resistance can be achieved by cleansing and abrading the scalp and taping electrodes filled with a conducting gel to the prepared surface. The more traditional technique from EEG laboratories involves abrading through a perforated electrode after it is sealed to the skin or scalp with collodion. Collodion-fixed electrodes will remain stable for hours. The "pasting" technique requires less abrasion to the scalp and less equipment and will provide adequate resistance reduction for less time, 1 to 2 hours generally. It is important to test the electrodes for adequate reduction of skin resistance to 3000 to 5000 ohms or less. Also, balancing of interelectrode resistance is important in eliminating large differences as well as attempting to gain low impedances to make CMR effective.[15] However, under adverse conditions we have recorded responses from electrodes at 9000 ohms, but we have also balanced resistance among the electrodes.

Pitfalls

There are some other special considerations with electrode placement. The following suggestions are based on our experience with more than 6000 recordings in the course of which a number of pitfalls were encountered.

1. *Reference placement problems.* There are some practical considerations in choosing the reference location. Old mastoid bowls are poor sites, both because of difficulty in attaching the electrode cup to the pitted area and because of comparatively poor conductivity of the underlying tissue. Scarred or keratomatous earlobes are also poor conductors. In both cases an alternative site is recommended.

2. *Protection from the transducer.* If the earspeaker is employed, it may dislodge the electrode, particularly if it is placed on the outside surface of the earlobe. Placing it on the mastoid process or the mesial surface of the earlobe generally provides the protection of the pinna when the earphone is in place. The mesial surface of the earlobe is more neutral and is not in direct contact with the transducer cover; it is also less comfortable and occasionally cannot be tolerated long enough to complete the procedure.

3. *Access for placement.* The front surface of the pinna provides easy access even on a sleeping or anesthetized patient. The tissue has relatively low natural resistance, although the electrodes are occasionally dislodged by contact with the earphone cushions.

4. *Patient artifacts.* If scar tissue is present at the active electrode site, placement should be varied to accommodate or avoid it. Of course the active electrode provides unacceptable contact if attached through a toupee, but there will also be excessive resistance over a hair transplant. A plastic surgical prosthesis increases resistance to potential transfer, and a prosthesis creates a huge artifact. In one patient, evaluation of asymmetrical hearing loss went on for more than an hour without obtaining proper recording conditions before the patient mentioned that he had a right temporal bone prosthesis. We obtained ABR measurements by using neck tissue on both sides with the anticipated but manageable neuromuscular artifact introduced by this placement. Another potential problem is scalp dandruff or psoriasis; psoriatic detritus is a distinctly poor electric conductor. It is advisable to clean the area carefully with a cosmetic sponge to reach the scalp and provide a good electrode field. In general, electrode placement should accommodate any special patient problems to provide low scalp-skin resistance and roughly equal interelectrode balance.

Patient State

The next step in administering ABR is to provide a good test environment. The primary consideration is the subject's state of relaxation. Generally, adults will cooperate sufficiently to provide an ongoing EEG on the order of 10^5 μv. If the environment is restful and the patient can lie down, the record will generally be quiet enough. Because of the monotony of the click stimuli, many subjects will sleep, providing ideal recording conditions. Although it is certainly helpful to test the patient in quiet, because noise will reduce response amplitude and make patient relaxation more difficult, room noise like that of an intensive care unit or surgical theater does not preclude successful suprathreshold administration of the test.

Response latencies are not affected by depth of sleep, sedation, anesthesia, or by any other drug at nontoxic levels. Starr and Achor[16] reported excellent clinical results even with patients in drug coma, and Stockard and Jones[17] found effects of drug or anesthesia only at massive doses. In particular the anticonvulsants at therapeutic levels had no effects. Tranquilizers, including the families of phenothiazenes, benzodiazipines, and short-acting barbiturates, had no effect even at toxic doses (in cats). In several cases of toxic doses in humans, only one patient showed abnormal response, but his hypothermia was considered to be a critical factor affecting latency.[17] Steroids and antimicrobials even at mass doses in cats had no effect. Squires and colleagues[18] found that alcohol (ethanol) intoxication may prolong central conduction time in cats; data for humans are not available. Stockard and Jones[17] also reported that neither isoflurane nor barbiturates abolished brainstem responses when administered concentrations were well above levels maintained for a deep level of anesthesia. Enflurane did not abolish the response, but for unknown reasons later response components were affected selectively during the recovery phase. Other investigators have also reported no drug effect. Davis[1] has reported clinical use of secobarbital without effect, Stockard and Rossiter[9] have described patients with diazepam-induced relaxation, and Jerger and colleagues[5] have reported good results with chloral hydrate. Halothane (fluoranc) anesthesia has been used with children in our population and has provided normal central conduction time in 10 to 12 patients who required anesthesia for the procedure. One of the two patients with apparent abnormality had no response at all and subsequent polytomography revealed abnormal cochlear structure. A second patient had prolonged conduction from wave I to wave V and had several other indications of brainstem abnormality. Based on literature and our own experience, halothane anesthesia provides an excellent recording condition without biasing response characteristics. Ketamine is also popular in some sections of the country for anesthesia with pediatric patients, although there are undocumented reports that the agent can affect response. Because the drug sometimes has undesirable side effects in children, primarily in terms of its hallucinogenic nature, our anesthesiologists do not suggest its use routinely.

It is important to stress that drugs are seldom needed to obtain the desired response, but the patient can be tested under the influence of drugs, conscious or unconscious, with minimal effect on early auditory responses.

Some patients with neuromuscular disorders, arthritis, or anxiety will require special relaxation techniques. For straightforward psychological or physical tension, the physician may choose to administer a muscle relaxant or sedative. In rare cases, allowing the patient to submit to testing seated instead of in the customary supine position will provide adequate relaxation. Certainly, poor test response calls for a thorough analysis of test conditions. A 28-year-old female who presented with multiple otologic complaints, including hearing loss and vertigo, appeared apprehensive but cooperative during attempts to obtain auditory evoked responses. At the beginning of each measurement the patient response was quiet, but marked break-up consistent with neuromuscular activity eventually interrupted the run. The patient was requested to relax and maintain a quiet state, but with no improvement in the recording. On close observation we noted that the patient repeatedly dropped her head to the right shoulder and could not prevent this chronic sagging. Diazepam was administered and the subsequently obtained evoked potentials were found to be normal, although the patient was in the early stages of a neuromuscular disease of unknown etiology. Figure 3–5 indicates the difference between premedication and postmedication evoked potentials on the right ear.

Pediatric and uncooperative patients pose another challenge in creating a good test environment. Most children, even infants, can be tested if the examiner is patient and flexible with them. Some, however, do not provide reliable recordings in a reasonable amount of time without sedation. Although an audiologist may consider the need for sedation or anesthesia, decisions about how much and what kind must be made by a physician. Since patients who are hard to test are either often very young (less than age 3 years) or have multiple physical problems, the potential for adverse response may well increase in this group, compared to the average subject receiving the same dose. For this reason, it is strongly recommended that such special test conditions as sedation or drug-induced sleep be provided when an attending physician and emergency equipment are available. In our experience one subject with a functional

Figure 3–5. Two representative runs on a patient in chronic muscle spasm. Upper curves (without sedation) are difficult to analyze and present poor retest. Lower waveforms show responses (normal) from this same patient after oral administration of diazepam.

component to his hearing loss had to be sedated for ABR because he gritted his teeth for the initial test session. Sedation was ordered by the physician and shortly after administration (intramuscular and oral), it was possible to establish the degree of peripheral deficit in the high frequencies with a good retest. It should be stressed that the decision to provide sedatives was medical and that it was administered when constant supervision against potential adverse reactions was present.

Before drugs are considered, the clinician should attempt to obtain ABR without them, even with a pediatric subject. Infants will sleep if a parent can delay their nap time for the procedure and bring a hungry child to the test suite with bottle, blanket, and teddy bear or anything that will suggest naptime. Older children in the toddler category (roughly 12 to 36 months) may or may not cooperate in a reasonable amount of time. If a child in this age range cannot be assessed by more conventional techniques, it is possible that he also cannot relax adequately for reliable ABR. If they are to undergo other procedures such as radiological studies, general anesthesia for the combined procedures may be warranted. This application of ABR is warranted only in cases in which peripheral auditory response cannot be determined by other procedures. This application will be discussed in detail in Chapter 4.

In summary, although most patients will provide good response without special techniques, it is sometimes necessary to sedate or anesthetize the patient. The response is unaffected by patient state.

Repetition Rate

Repetition rate is a significant instrumentation variable. Site-of-lesion studies are obtained at a relatively slow repetition rate (20 pulses per second or less). Our laboratory uses 8 pulses per second for routine studies. Table 3-2 samples several reports of ABR for repetition rate. Repetition rate is important because an adequate interstimulus interval is necessary for baseline recording. Eggermont and colleagues[20] found the eighth nerve

TABLE 3–2. Repetition Rate Suggested in Various ABR Laboratories

Repetition Rate	
Selters and Brackmann[6]	20 pps
Stockard and Rossiter[9]	10 pps
Starr and Hamilton[10]	10 per sec
Mokotoff et al.[8]	33.3
Jerger et al.[3]	20
Davis[1]	20
Glasscock et al.[12]	8
Coats and Martin[4]	20
Fria and Sabo[19]	10 to 30 pps
Starr and Achor[10]	8

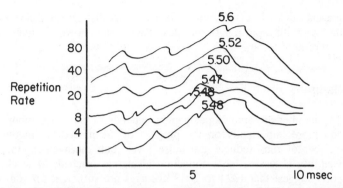

Figure 3–6. Illustration of increasing repetition rate for ABR with normal subject. Note both latency shift and loss of detail at high rates. N = 1024, I = 85 peSPL with 0.1 msec click.

action potential was markedly affected as the interstimulus interval was shortened below critical refractory period. Figure 3–6 illustrates the problems related to data collection at rapid repetition rates. This normal subject demonstrates responses consistent with the report by Weber and Fujikawa,[21] who found that repetition rate significantly affects intensity-latency functions in normal subjects. Theoretically, pathologic ears should also show changes as rate increases, but the patterns are not well documented. For clinical purposes it is important to use a sufficiently slow repetition rate so that the response is easily observed and subject to retest. The increase in test time at a slow rate is warranted in view of the more repeatable latency and improved detail of the response. However, faster repetition rates are useful in expediting threshold testing since a restless infant can be screened by rapid stimulation during the quiet periods that are available. The examiner can screen for wave V at fast rates, up to 40 pulses per second, although once the threshold can be estimated slow runs are necessary to extract the lower-amplitude wave V.

There are also reports using very rapid stimulus repetition to look at adaptation of evoked potentials. As demonstrated in Figure 3–7, responses in a normal subject show change in latency. As suggested by Thornton and Coleman's data,[22] a normal subject will demonstrate a latency increase adaptation apparently by cumulative loss at low and relatively high brainstem levels. There is the suggestion by Daly and colleagues[23] that an increase in repetition rate will aid in defining auditory pathology. Josey[24] reports that this rate abnormality occurs frequently in patients with eighth nerve tumors, although not in all of these subjects. Gerling and Finitzo[25] found changes at high repetition rates to be the only parameter reflecting abnormality in patients with documented central nervous system pathology and recommend routine inclusion of rapid rates in the test battery. The application of such techniques to documented pathology at varying levels of the auditory system is necessary before such data can be incorporated into routine clinical procedure. At present, there is insufficient information to distinguish the level of pathology with rapid repetition rates. These rates, however, may be useful in threshold tests.

Size of Sample

The number of samples per patient depends in part on computer design and more importantly on the purpose of the procedure. Increasing the number of runs reduces the noise level, but improvement in response visibility is less as large collection levels are reached. Most clinical reports suggest that 1024 to 2048 averages are sufficient for site-of-lesion procedures, whereas others use as many as 4000. Some of the variations are summarized in Table 3–3. In threshold testing the average needs to continue only long enough to determine the latency of wave V. At high intensity under good conditions this response may be evident after only 256 sweeps. Threshold procedures should vary the number of samples to obtain adequate response as efficiently as possible. As the intensity approaches the threshold, more samples are required to determine wave V latency than at suprathreshold levels. For this reason, samples at suspected threshold should include a relatively large average, at least 1024. For most clinical applications 2048 runs reach the upper limit of practical reduction of noise through repetition, and 1024 are often sufficient.

Stimulus Intensity

Stimulus intensity is another important variable. Peak latency of wave V is not achieved until 40 to 60 dB above threshold. Response amplitude may increase with intensity growth, but latency will not diminish above this point. As intensity is decreased, wave V latency will increase until threshold is reached (Fig. 3–7). Wave V is the most persistent auditory brainstem response and is still recordable near voluntary threshold, whereas recording of the entire Jewett sequence requires suprathreshold testing. There is also a marked improvement in amplitude with increased intensity. Some site-of-lesion reports[6,9,16] suggest sampling at one intensity

TABLE 3–3. Number of Samples Per Run Suggested in Several ABR Laboratories

Reference	Samples per Average
Selters and Brackmann[6]	1000
Mokotoff et al.[8]	1024 to 4096
Stockard and Rossiter[9]	2000 to 4000
Starr and Hamilton[10]	2048
Coats and Martin[4]	1000
Glasscock et al.[12]	1000

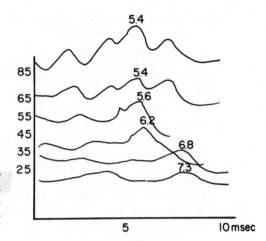

Figure   3–7. Latency-intensity function in a normal-hearing subject. As intensity is increased, amplitude increases and latency decreases.

only. Others[12,26] vary intensity according to degree of loss. Central conduction time is easier to analyze at a relatively loud presentation level (roughly 40 to 60 dB over stimulus threshold), but identification is severely complicated near threshold. Hayes[27] found that severe hearing loss in the 1000–4000 Hz range prevented unambiguous ABR interpretation in 13 (22%) of 60 cases of confirmed eighth nerve lesions. Interpretation of site-of-lesion tests based on latency of wave V without regard to sensation level of the signal runs the risk of unnecessary false-positive response readings. The stimulus must provoke high-frequency response to provide sufficient synchrony for a visible wave V. Practically speaking, the sound must be above action potential threshold by a minimum of 40 dB in a normal system to reach the most efficient wave V. For a patient with high-frequency loss, interpretation of the averaged response at arbitrary stimulation level is unnecessarily difficult. The sound intensity should be manipulated to accommodate hearing loss, so that sufficient data are available to evaluate central conduction time or at least to determine whether an increase in intensity will decrease the latency of wave V. The alternative is to hold intensity constant[6] and to interpret the latency of wave V with regard to the degree of loss with a formula based on clinical findings of proven cochlear lesions of known loss.

In our clinical use of ABR we have adopted a guideline for applying ABR interpretation to severe hearing loss subjects when only wave V is presented. It is based in part on Sanders'[28] report that ABRs most closely predict the 1000–4000 Hz average threshold. If the 1000–4000 Hz pure tone average is poorer than 75 dB nHL, the patient response must include a wave V latency within normal limits, or it must contain waves I, III, and V for interpeak conduction time interpolation. If the 1000–4000 Hz average loss is poorer than 75 dB, wave V is delayed, and interpeak intervals cannot be calculated, then the ABR is compromised as a test for site of lesion. This guideline does not prevent attempts at gathering ABR data in patients with more severe loss. Occasionally recruiting ears will provide enough of the Jewett sequence to allow the examiner to evaluate the retrocochlear pathways.

Generally site-of-lesion evaluation should begin at a relatively loud level (40 to 60 dB above average threshold for the stimulus in normal subjects). For site-of-lesion test patients, the audiogram will allow a prediction of required stimulus intensity or will suggest possible compromise of test interpretation because of the severity of the loss. Since the test stimulus is not a standard audiometric signal, it is useful to establish voluntary threshold for the test stimulus. When patient thresholds for the stimuli are not obtainable, the formula and statistical data of Selters and Brackmann[6] and Jerger and colleagues[5] provide an indirect interpolation of acceptable latency of wave V. If wave I can also be determined, central conduction time will make retrocochlear site-of-lesion test interpretation independent of stimulus intensity. Variation of intensity in 10 dB steps from threshold to earliest wave V latency will also yield a latency-intensity function that is helpful in separating conductive from cochlear lesions, as will be described in Chapter 4. Steep latency functions are consistent with cochlear disorder,[5] whereas functions that are displaced but parallel to normal represent conductive hearing loss.

A latency-intensity curve is also established in threshold testing. Because wave amplitude is a function of stimulus intensity, it is advisable to begin the procedure well above the estimated threshold, where wave V is relatively easy to identify. The threshold of wave V in ideal test conditions is also highly repeatable, although it is much smaller in amplitude, and latency is increased (Fig. 3–8).

Preamplifier Filters

Filter settings also affect the auditory responses, most prominently in amplitude. Many clinicians agree on 3000 Hz as the high-frequency setting because there is relatively little significant information above that frequency range, but noise in the recording is somewhat increased (Fig. 3–8). There is much less agreement on low-frequency setting because there is a significant increase in noise as the setting is lowered (Fig. 3–9). Because the auditory responses vary in latency and morphology as the low-frequency cut-off is changed, it is important to maintain a constant low-frequency setting for comparison of the patient response to normal subjects in interpreting evoked potentials. For example, changing the filter from 50 to 300 Hz to eliminate noise will preclude interpreting wave V latency in terms of the normative data established at 50 Hz. It is helpful to filter out low-frequency noise in difficult situations such as testing in an intensive care unit, but the examiner must be aware that the response is biased. Ordinarily, an effectively quiet recording can be obtained with a low-frequency filter setting of 50 or 100 Hz. In summary, filters should be varied to accommodate the test environment, but re-

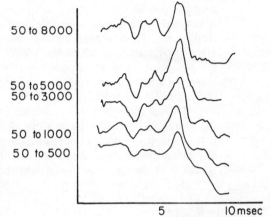

Figure 3–8. Effect of altering high-frequency filter for auditory evoked potentials on a normal-hearing subject. Low-pass setting is held constant at 50 Hz. Detail is distorted at 1 kHz and lower, but little is added as filter is set above 3 kHz. (1024 samples at 85 peSPL, 0.1 msec click).

sponse interpretation should be documented by a knowledge of normal responses with those filter settings.

Stimulus Characteristics

The stimulus must have a rapid rise time and high-frequency energy to provoke a synchronous discharge. Some clinical stimulus generators allow the examiner to vary signal characteristics. For site-of-lesion procedures, the high-frequency brief duration settings provide maximal amplitude with more precise wave peaks, making the recording easier to analyze. At frequencies below 1000 Hz the tone stimulates a relatively broad segment of the basilar membrane toward the apical turn of the cochlea, with the result that the desynchronous response is difficult or impossible to analyze reliably.[1] This procedure does not allow for sampling response through the entire frequency range for hearing, but it is possible to obtain

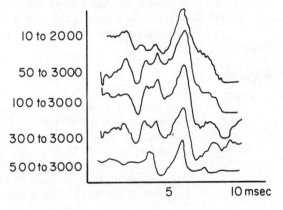

Figure 3–9. Effect of altering low-frequency filter for auditory evoked potentials on a normal-hearing subject. High-pass setting is held constant at 3000 Hz. Noise increases significantly at 50 Hz and lower. However, response detail is somewhat better at 100 Hz and lower (1024 samples, 85 peSPL, 0.1 msec).

averages with the stimulus frequency range approximating 1000 Hz. Wave V thresholds are not as repeatable at low frequency as they are in higher ranges, nor do they approximate voluntary thresholds as closely as at higher frequencies, at which the wave V threshold is highly retestable at an average of 10 dB over voluntary threshold for normal subjects. Alternative methods for inferring the low-frequency threshold have been tried and are reviewed in Chapter 4.

Because different types of stimuli are in use, it is important to define the stimulus as precisely as possible. Specifying the electric impulse only is not completely adequate because the transducer modification is generally considerable. The stimulus is defined much better if the acoustic spectrum of the signal is also presented.

Stimulus Phase

Another signal characteristic that affects the response is stimulus phase. Alternating polarity will eliminate the early electrical and mechanical artifacts in averaging along with the CM, although it will not affect the compound action potential. However, averaging both condensation and rarefaction waves will have the effect of desynchronizing the response because these two phases will have slightly different timing in stimulating the cochlea. There is a small error or variation in wave latency in comparing rarefaction with condensation stimuli, since this phase shift will cause a slightly different generation of the action potential and may or may not be apparent upon averaging, depending on the nature of the time-lock of stimulus and averager. Coats and Martin[4] found that in high-frequency loss rarefaction responses were out of phase with condensation runs at waves II through IV, whereas there was little difference at wave V. They suggest that there are two components in the response, that is, two parallel pathways, with waves III, IV, and VI representing one pathway and wave V a different route. Schwartz and Berry[29] recommend the rarefaction click because of the increased amplitude and improved resolution of wave I. Pending further clinical investigation as to the origin of this difference, the important factor here is to settle on a consistent choice of polarity to eliminate this additional source of variation.

Masking

The use of masking to prevent crossover of the stimulus to the nontest ear is standard protocol for most test procedures. Masking is also important in determining whether the right or left pathways are under test in evoked response audiometry. Masking desynchronizes response of the opposite ear to minimize its contribution. Interaural attenuation is relatively large, roughly 60 dB for a stimulus exciting regions higher than 3000 Hz, which is the range of most site-of-lesion stimuli. Whether contralateral masking is present or not, off-side responses should be suspected when markedly abnormal patterns are present. If a crossover response appears, its latencies should be those of stimuli approximately 60 dB lower than the intensity to the opposite ear. Remarkably, this crossover is not always seen. Further studies are certainly needed to define masking more precisely.

If the response is off-side, amplitude will be comparatively poor. Suppose, for instance, the clinician knows nothing about the patient, presents the clicks to the right ear, and obtains a threshold of 20 dB peSPL at 0.1 msec. If the opposite ear yields no response until 90 dB at 8.2 msec, is the wave crossover or representative of left ear response? Desynchronizing the opposite ear with masking in this case will eliminate participation of the off-side ear. It may also damp the amplitude of the target response somewhat. When possible crossover problems complicate data interpretation, the clinician may want to consider impedance audiometry, ECochG, or ABR with bone-conducted stimuli (See Chap. 5).

Patient Variables

Amplitude and latency are somewhat sex-dependent. Stockard and colleagues[30] recommend maintaining latency data by sex for close examination of responses. In reviewing ABR for 20 young female and 20 young male subjects (less than age 30 years) in our group, the mean latency of wave V was 0.15 msec later in men, although there was overlap in the ranges. Jerger and Hall[31] found latency in both normal hearing and hearing-impaired female subjects to be significantly shorter (about 0.2 msec) than that of men. Further analysis of the test variable is needed to confirm this tendency. Sex may also influence amplitude, since this measure has been described as larger in the young female.[30] Certainly it is easy to demonstrate a dramatic Jewett wave V on a young cooperative female. In a review of 20 male and 20 female patients with normal responses in our clinic, amplitude was compared by measuring voltage from maximum positive to maximum negative in waves I, III, and V. Although wave I and wave III amplitudes were virtually interchangeable in comparing the two groups, wave V averaged 12.7 percent larger for females than for those in the male group, with a range of −4.0 percent to a 32 percent increase. Although this description is insufficient to confirm evoked-potential sex differences, it does suggest that the reports of such differences in amplitude have some merit and deserve further consideration. Because of its retest variability, amplitude has received less attention than latency.

Age-related variations in amplitude and intensity have also been reported. Hecox and Galambos[32] found that wave V latency was prolonged at birth and that maturation to adult response time occurred primarily by 12 months. Their infant data show latency as a function of age, making it clear that the clinician must take into account the neural maturation of the patient. In fact, because wave V latencies may be no earlier at suprathreshold than 8 to 9 msec in the first few weeks of life, including premature birth, response acquisition requires a longer dwell time (up to 20 msec) than the normally recommended gate of 10 msec for brainstem responses.

The data of Mokotoff and co-workers[8] included premature infants and demonstrated that response latency is a function of gestational age. The reasons for the delay are not fully established, although the data suggest normal changes in myelin as well as maturation of the auditory system. Galambos has also indicated that absorption of mesenchime in the neonate is slow and this material provides a conductive block to the sound.[32] The delay is not a simple conductive disorder, since central conduction times are also prolonged in comparison to normal subjects. Amplitude may be greater in infants because it is easier to establish low electrode resistance and the connecting tissues are more efficient conductors. In general, wave V responses are large in amplitude, making them highly visible and reliable for interpretation.[30] In adults, there is tendency for latency to increase with age greater than 50.

In our own review of central conduction time in 14 females age 60 to 74 years, with essentially normal hearing (threshold 25 dB to 40 dB hearing level [HL] at 4000 and 8000 Hz), there was no significant difference in wave V latency in comparison with younger adults. A male group of 10 ears with essentially normal audiologic responses presented a mean wave V latency 0.3 msec greater than that of young normal subjects, with prolongation spread over the entire series of waves and not confined to upper or lower brainstem responses. The range of these men for wave I to wave V conduction time was greater than for younger men, since two subjects had latencies well within normal limits. These results do not prove a latency shift in the aging population, but they do suggest the need to investigate average latency in the geriatric population. Until further documentation is available, we assume that aging affects both ears symmetrically in auditory conduction, so that geriatric patients at the upper limits of normal range of latency serve as their own control. More emphasis should be placed on interaural differences in this instance than on statistically normal wave V latency with these patients.

Stockard and co-workers[30] described variations in response secondary to hypothermia, in which reduced body temperature was found to prolong conduction time slightly. Although such patients are infrequently seen, they may be found among drug overdose and comatose subjects. For this reason clinicians should consider this factor in the analysis of potential hypothermia subjects, even though there is insufficient data to predict latency in a known hypothermic patient. Significant temperature-related effects may occur in the presence of demyelinating disease. A neurologic history of multiple sclerosis patients often reveals exacerbation of symptoms when the patient is hot and perspiring but amelioration of symptoms with cooling. We performed ABR on a patient with multiple sclerosis at 60°F and then at 80°F with the patient in thermal blankets

Figure 3–10. Responses for a 28-year-old female with multiple sclerosis. Condition A at 60°F room temperature approaches normal with good retest. Condition B at 80°F suggests a decrease in retest. The figure includes three binaural averages for both conditions.

A 60°

B 80°

5   IOmsec

and complaining of overheating. The patient's body temperature was not obtained because this was only an attempt to determine whether ABR could document this patient's complaint. As demonstrated in Figure 3–10, the wave morphology approached normal under cool conditions but showed markedly poor retest with the patient complaining of being uncomfortably warm.

Because response acquisition is the result of appropriate instrumentation and technique, it is important to leave the protocol flexible and in the hands of a skilled and insightful clinician. "Cookbook" approaches are helpful, but following rigid procedures will result in insufficient response data, particularly when abnormal auditory systems are being evaluated. The clinician who encounters unusual responses must be sufficiently sophisticated to manipulate stimulus variables to try to confirm the nature of the auditory abnormality and to rule out error in instrumentation.

Response Interpretation

Response interpretation primarily involves analysis of latency and amplitude. Although both vary with stimulus sensation level, latency is a highly retestable sequence; amplitude is markedly less so. For most clinical applications, the emphasis is on the latency of the waves. Because stimulus characteristics affect latency, each laboratory needs to establish its own normative data. At suprathreshold level, wave V latency is on the order of 5 to 6 msec, with each preceding wave about 1 msec earlier. However, there is a very small range for normal adult response to a given signal, on the order of 0.4 msec for most commonly used stimuli. The exceptions for sex and age have already been described. To interpret the data with such precision, clinicians must define the normal range for their own technique and stimulus.

How does one report the results? First, the test interpretation is shaped by the purpose of the procedure. If threshold assessment is the object, wave V latency increases are monitored as intensity is decreased. At some intensity level, the latency for a wave V will be approximately 8 to 9 msec, with repeatability. With a 10 dB decrease beyond this, there will be no recordable, retestable bump in the averaged EEG. Threshold for wave V is commonly defined as the lowest intensity at which the response is visible in the recording. This technique will allow a threshold search as well as a plot of latency versus intensity. For high-frequency sounds, the threshold for wave V is highly retestable under good conditions. It is approximately 10 dB above the voluntary threshold for perception of the signal in normal-hearing adults. It is important to remember that signals approaching 1000 Hz produce poorer retest results, with responses visible only at approximately 30 dB above threshold by routine audiometry. Interpretation of ABR thresholds should incorporate not only comment on the actual threshold of the response but also awareness of the relationship of its significance in terms of a normal response.

Site-of-lesion analysis is generally attempted for suprathreshold averages and should consist of comparison of interwave latencies I to V. Although the label of central conduction may not be altogether technically accurate for the wave I to wave V travel time, it is a useful term in describing results. Because this index looks at responses above threshold in the cochlea, in effect it eliminates so-called delay resulting from inner ear pathology. If central conduction time is not considered, interpretation of delay in the latency of wave V must include a possible delay in brainstem conduction, an elevated threshold of response in the cochlea, or an attenuation in the form of middle ear disease. In such situations wave V responses can be interpreted only in the face of other information about the auditory system. For example, a clinician testing a comatose patient with head injuries and with no other information available may obtain a wave V at 7 msec from both sides at 85 peSPL. How should such responses be interpreted? Could they represent cochlear deficit? The patient could have experienced considerable vascular distress or may have a prior history of sensorineural loss. Do they represent a massive brainstem lesion? Too little is known at this point to make a definite interpretation. The clinician should then look for central conduction time. If wave I is found at 3.8 msec in both ears, the clinician is now able to report normal central conduction time at this level and can begin to suspect that the patient's response is the result of attenuation at the middle ear or cochlea. One can further enhance the interpretation with latency-intensity functions and bone-conduction responses. Conversely, suppose this comatose patient presents a normal latency of wave I in both ears. Since wave I to wave V conduction is prolonged, the clinician may now look to the auditory nerve and brainstem for the problem. One may even find that by looking at wave I to wave II, wave II to wave III, and each successive interval one is able to speculate more precisely about the level of the auditory breakdown. Although central conduction time or some variant of this index is not universally reported, several authors have found it a sensitive tool.[6,12,16]

Straightforward comparison of absolute wave V latency against mean and range for wave V is also sensitive though less reflective of site of auditory breakdown. With absolute latency comparisons, the examiner must be careful to take into account the possibility of asymmetrical peripheral loss resulting in differences in latency between ears. Because wave V latency decreases as suprathreshold stimulus intensity increases, the examiner must take the latency intensity function under consideration. For example, a subject may present a voluntary threshold for the click stimulus that is 50 dB poorer in the impaired ear than in the opposite ear. The procedure was run at 70 dB above the good ear threshold so that the response reflected normal latency from the good side, but with only a 20-dB sensation level (SL) to the impaired ear wave V was delayed by comparison. Clearly this test is biased by differences in the stimulation sensation level, and any comparison of absolute latency of wave V will reflect it. The impaired ear response could wrongly be interpreted as a central delay when it is in fact only an averaged response at a low sensation level. If the patient voluntary or ABR threshold suggests severe reduction in sensitivity, absolute latency data comparisons cannot be made without other information. Alternatives include (1) assessment of latency-intensity functions to compare ears at an equal sensation level above wave V threshold, (2) increase in stimulus intensity (if possible) to yield a wave V at its earliest possible latency in that ear, and (3) aborting the procedure in favor of other special tests that can be interpreted even with severe loss present. With caution, analysis of latency of wave V is a useful index for interpreting ABR responses.

Interaural comparisons are also useful in response analysis. Because variations related to sex, age, and other factors should have a symmetric effect, any difference between ears is thought to suggest breakdown in the auditory pathways on the slower side. Selters and Brackmann[6] have found this to be a sensitive comparison for these subjects. In our own experience, interaural comparison of central conduction time from waves I to V is an excellent tool for reducing the rate of misinterpretation, primarily because it eliminates the bias in difference in peripheral sensitivity.

Latency-intensity functions also provide assistance in analysis of the site of the lesion. Separation of cochlear deficit from conductive loss can be enhanced by consideration of latency-intensity chances.[5,32] If the latency of wave V is plotted as a function of intensity, the normal subject will yield a curve ranging about 3 msec from threshold to about 50 dB SL. The conductive loss will yield a function parallel to the normal, but the conductive lesion will be displaced by the amount of the loss. In cochlear lesions the curve steepens, so that less intensity increase is needed to achieve the earliest latency of wave V. We have observed this phenomenon only when there is high-frequency hearing loss, thus often excluding "early" Meniere's disease. In 73 ears assessed by latency functions with clinical diagnosis of cochlear disorder, primarily Meniere's disease, the mean threshold for the click response was 53.3 peSPL (range 35 to 75 dB); that is, 86.3 percent were found to have a steep latency-intensity function, whereas 13.7 percent had displaced but otherwise normal curves. Although in our series a steep latency-intensity function was seen only in cochlear pathology conditions, not all cochlear ears had steep functions. Some patients with sensorineural loss exhibit normal latency-intensity functions, possibly reflecting differences related to types of cochlear disorder. Latency-intensity functions help to document the site of the lesion, but care must be taken to support interpretation by other techniques such as impedance audiometry.

In comparison to the relatively precise application of latency interpretation, close amplitude evaluations are more difficult to make. This is so because of the relative amplitude of the various waves among normal subjects, and retest amplitudes vary considerably more than retest latencies. Interpolation of absolute amplitude is also more difficult because baselines float and retest produces variation; however, such gross variations as noted by Stockard and Rossiter[9] are clinically useful observations. There are patients whose wave I amplitude will be markedly large— for example, in comparison to normal range and other responses in that ear. In our experience, morphologic variants of a gross nature are often followed by deterioration in the remaining waves. Musiek and associates[33] report that a wave I–wave V ratio of less than 1.00 seldom occurred in normal or cochlear ears but was seen in 44 percent of their retrocochlear subjects. A normal variation is an increase in wave V response amplitude of about 75 percent with binaural stimulation if the signal intensity is above threshold bilaterally. There is some suggestion that failure to achieve such amplitude increase with binaural stimulation represents abnormality in the upper brainstem. Figure 3–11 demonstrates this relatively subtle abnormality in a subject with multiple sclerosis. Explanations for such changes are only speculative but theoretically may reflect the breakdown of monitoring or feedback in the presence of a massive disorder of the auditory pathways. Gross variations in amplitude help document abnormality even though we do not understand fully the mechanisms involved. As technique is improved, closer monitoring of amplitude range should sharpen the clinical interpretation of ABR responses.

In summary, response analysis consists of consideration of latency and amplitude. Because of high reliability, latency relations can be in-

Figure 3–11. Responses from a patient with multiple sclerosis. Right and left ear responses show slight prolongation at waves III to V. Binaural test does not result in the normal amplitude increase (represented by the dotted line). Sample 1K, 8 pps, 85 dB peSPL, 0.1 msec (filtered click).

spected closely for wave V latency, wave-to-wave conduction times, and interaural differences in latency. Gross variations from normal in amplitude should also be noted.

RESPONSE REPORTING

Because the clinician must be prepared to share test results with colleagues in a variety of disciplines, it is important to make the interpretation relevant to the patient's overall diagnosis and rehabilitative program. The report should compare the brainstem responses to predicted behavioral thresholds, with care to point out the critical limitations of this technique. The threshold responses should be reported for wave V but not in any way as representing the same auditory capacity indicated by volunteered thresholds for pure tones. Likewise, the site-of-lesion report should be as specific to point of breakdown as reasonable with the caveat that each wave in the sequence does not directly reflect a specific nucleus. The responses will provide evidence sometimes consistent with conductive disorder, or in other instances with cochlear pathology, eighth nerve or low brainstem breakdown, and so on. It is possible to attempt to be more specific in assigning the site of lesion than present data will permit. The wise clinician will also avoid any attempt at diagnosis of the abnormality, since any response variation may be caused by one of several pathologic conditions. One patient complaining of bilateral tinnitus was referred after an apparent delay in wave V was thought to represent a bilateral eighth nerve lesion. A subsequent work-up revealed severe high-frequency sensorineural loss bilaterally with normal central conduction on ABR at a higher intensity than in the earlier test. A myelogram was performed with no evidence of a space-occupying lesion. Special tests were otherwise consistent with a cochlear pathologic condition bilaterally (by history, noise-induced loss).

The test report should also be helpful in providing some information about conditions because there is no standard protocol for testing. Other clinicians need to know the test conditions, including the type of stimulus, the repetition rate, the number of samples per average, the stimulus intensity, the retest reliability of the response, whether the patient is sedated or awake, and the basis for defining abnormal response. Only in this manner can consideration to repeating or documenting results be given, until such time as some of these variables are specified in a commonly accepted protocol.

In summary, attempting to define the kind of lesion with ABR is a serious abuse of the test. In addition, interpretation of ABR without any other data, whether subjective or in the form of other procedures such as routine audiometry of impedance audiometry or whatever protocol is possible, is an unwarranted gamble. Seldom are all tests except ABR precluded. Interpreting responses must be based on the framework of documentation by other audiologic procedures, ABR retest, and other clinical information, including the patient's history.

CALIBRATION TECHNIQUE

The clinician should monitor equipment output as part of routine maintenance. Much of the maintenance has to do with verifying timer characteristics, average performance, and other technical considerations that can be monitored by the manufacturer or by someone trained in computer electronics. The stimulus, however, should be monitored at the test site for the same reasons that a standard audiometer requires a calibration check. Determining sound pressure level (SPL) output is not as straightforward as a routine audiometer output check, because the stimuli are brief in duration. If a sound level meter with impulse capture is available, output at the transducer can be observed. Alternatively peSPL can be determined by displaying the signal on an oscilloscope and noting the peak-to-peak amplitude. With the same set-up, a known pure tone is driven through the transducer (generally at the resonant frequency of the earphone) and adjusted to provide the same peak-to-peak amplitude as the test stimulus on the oscilloscope. The SPL required to match amplitude as indicated at the SPL meter is the peak equivalent SPL of the stimulus. Either of these techniques will provide a reference for monitoring output, since there is minimal information standardizing specification of click or brief-tone intensity. In addition, biological calibration between laboratory checks will help to monitor changes in output. Normal threshold for click can be established with a normal "jury" of 5 or 10 subjects as used in our clinic to provide a basis for biological calibration.

Another consideration in calibration is monitoring for any changes in frequency response. Stimulus shape should be defined when new equipment is received. If periodic comparisons are to be of a significant documentation change, the clinician must monitor not only the electric impulse but also the acoustic form of the signal through the transducer to be used in the clinic. Otherwise important considerations such as rise time and peak stimulus frequency will not be adequately included in interpretation of the section of the auditory system under test. Generator or transducer malfunction can rarely be "heard" even by the so-called trained listener. For this reason acoustic output should be included as part of the calibration procedure.

REVIEW OF TEST TECHNIQUE

The following sections are a review with emphasis on suggestions of test protocol, or a kind of "game plan." It is important to stress that the protocol must be flexible for the insightful clinician to capture as much information as possible about the auditory system of the individual. At the same time, the procedure is somewhat determined by the characteristics of the equipment being used for evoking the potentials.

The plan is determined by the nature of the primary information being sought, roughly grouped as either threshold search or site-of-lesion test. If the purpose of the test is to obtain thresholds, the following guidelines are a good model to follow, although they are not a hard-and-fast plan. (The guidelines assume that the clinician has already obtained normative data with his/her equipment.)

Provide a quiet, relaxing setting with a couch or bed for supine testing. Before attempting to obtain a suitable test state, the electrodes should be applied. If a child is to nap, electrodes should be fixed with the electrode wires out of reach before the child relaxes, so there will be no need to arouse or antagonize children after they settle down. It also helps to feed children just prior to testing, and to provide them with a pillow or favorite blanket or anything else to suggest naptime. For some reason, perhaps boredom, a large number of subjects drowse or sleep during testing even though the first several averages may look noisy. For this reason we nearly always anticipate patient cooperation without the use of drugs. By affixing the electrodes immediately and attempting to acquire a response, we are generally able to achieve recordable responses. With infants it is sometimes necessary to introduce the signal with a hand-held earphone or mounted speaker until deep sleep is achieved.

If the aforementioned techniques do not satisfactorily prepare the patient and a repeatable wave cannot be measured, an artifact must be suspected. Although an absence of repeatable waves in an awake patient may reflect auditory problems, retest in a state of sleep will be necessary to validate the response. The supervising physician will determine the method of sedation based on patient age and health. With some subjects, such as very young or multiply handicapped patients, administration of general anesthesia to produce light sleep may be considered safer than the use of sedatives and has the further advantage of direct medical supervision. Because general anesthesia is usually administered in a hospital, the expense and potential risk should be balanced against the need for ABR. Generally, subjecting a child to medication would be contraindicated if auditory behavior could be observed and retested in the sound field. However, because ABR is an important technique in early identification of hearing loss, special procedures such as sedation may be warranted in otherwise difficult cases.

As an example, a Korean orphan aged 2.5 years came to the United States to be adopted by a military family. Only the adopting mother could control or relate to the child without a fear response from him. She suspected deafness as a complicating factor in his failure to communicate. The child also exhibited behavior suggestive of cultural shock and withdrawal, and as he had already experienced several temporary care settings, the team working with the family wanted to rule out hysterical deafness. This child spoke no Korean or English but did reportedly "chatter" while playing. Because of his shyness and withdrawal he alternated between a passive state and sobbing during testing, so that two different hearing clinics were unable to determine with any certainty the degree of hearing loss. Impedance audiometry failed to provide an estimate of the loss because of the child's constant sobbing during repeated tests. In view of the patient's history, the otologist ordered polytomography, a procedure requiring anesthesia for most children less than 7 years of age. While the child was anesthetized, we conducted ABR and impedance audiometry. Tympanometry suggested slight negative pressure with absent reflexes bilaterally. No response was obtained for ABR at maximum intensity. Based on two tests the patient was thought to have a severe auditory disorder. An external canal electrode was positioned next to the tympanic membrane but no N_1 response or action potential was observed, suggesting a severe peripheral deficit. If the child had not been drugged, the absence of response would have been inconclusive, making it the third audiologic evaluation unable to rule out or confirm hearing loss. Since the patient was in a monitored sleep state, results were labeled as consistent with a severe bilateral peripheral deficit. Polytomography immediately followed the auditory potential studies and revealed a marked abnormality of both cochleae, providing an unusual instance of immediate substantiation of ABR findings. The child is now in a program for deaf children specially adapted to his unusual language problems. In most cases it is important to continue attempts at traditional audiometry in order to analyze the subject's ability to process whatever sound is provided from the auditory periphery.

Although there are situations in which steps such as the use of anesthesia are warranted, for most patients sedation is sufficient. It is important to provide adequate medical supervision for such cases. For instance, hyperactive patients who cannot be tested by routine methods are quite likely to respond adversely to sedatives such as secobarbital and chloral hydrate. If the activity level increases, it only frustrates the examiner. If there is a shock response, emergency procedures may be necessary to prevent fatality. It is a good practice to suspect the patient's state when ABR results are not subject to reliable retest or are absent. Voluntary sleep represents the optimum patient state for testing. Failing this, medical supervision for drug-induced sleep or anesthesia is in order.

It is possible for an uncooperative subject to obstruct the test without the examiner's knowledge. In a test, for example, the patient can thwart testing by chronic neuromuscular contamination. The example demonstrated in Figure 3–12 was obtained by completing an average with the subject's jaw clenched on demand, with the resulting apparent response abnormality. In our experience wily patients can bias even such objective tests as impedance audiometry and ABR. It may be advisable to obtain sedation for such patients, again with care to ensure medical supervision.

To minimize the duration of the threshold test procedure, begin testing with binaural stimulation at a moderately high intensity, 90 dB peSPL. Using a rapid repetition rate such as 40 pulses per second, binaural stimulation will allow the examiner to scan for wave V threshold because it

Figure 3–12. Normal subject. Right ear tested during relaxation while subject deliberately clenched teeth for left ear stimulation. Sample 1024 at 8 pps, 60 dB SL (subject threshold), 0.1 msec filtered click.

has higher visibility with binaural search and persists even at high repetition rates. The determination of whether both ears are responding can be made by repeating the run stimulating only one side. If the response amplitude is unchanged, probably only one ear is participating; if it drops, both are contributing. For rapid searches, we stimulate binaurally at high repetition rates and relatively small samples (512), with a decrease in intensity until wave V cannot be observed. Near estimated threshold intensity, a large sample (at least 1000) with monaural stimulation at a slower rate (for example, 8 pps) is obtained, varying intensity in 10 dB steps to find the lowest intensity at which wave V can be detected. The same procedure is repeated contralaterally. Reproducibility is verified on retest; then, if possible, stimulus frequency characteristics are altered and the procedure is repeated. A control run with no stimulus to the earspeaker but all other conditions held constant should produce no response. If there is an apparent response, then either there is an instrumentation error, the patient is poorly relaxed, or there is a time-locked artifact. Such "responses" raise serious questions regarding interpretation of ABR thresholds in these patients.

For site-of-lesion testing, the technique must be modified. Best results are obtained with a slow repetition rate, generally less than ten per second with a relatively large sample (1000 or more) and suprathreshold stimulation. In contrast to threshold procedures, patient relaxation is important, but responses can generally be obtained from a quiet patient without requiring a sleep state. Latencies should be recorded, amplitude noted, and the procedure repeated. Latencies should be retestable at no more than 0.1 msec variation for tolerance in reading errors. If the runs do not overlap in latency, the responses cannot be considered reliable. The troubleshooting section that follows will suggest some techniques when retest results are poor. Some possibilities are poor test environment (including patient state), equipment artifact, or an active disease process such as multiple sclerosis. Generally, two trials are sufficient to prove retest, and the examiner can proceed directly to the contralateral ear. If the response appears abnormal it is wise to obtain an average under the same conditions but complete attenuation of the signal. A null or straight-line recording should result, indicating that the bumps in the preceding average reflected auditory response.

Starting with the better side in asymmetrical losses will help the examiner to assess a patient's response pattern for better comparison with the off-side response. If beginning the data collection at 90 peSPL does not provide a normal sequence, the intensity should be increased. As a rule, pure tone audiometry precedes site-of-lesion testing in our clinic. It helps to obtain threshold for the ABR stimulus also. When thresholds are available, intensity for testing can be chosen with little loss of test time. If voluntary threshold is known, the absence of wave V is interpreted more reliably, although the relationship between audibility of the stimulus and number of responders to evoke a synchronous discharge is unknown. In general, when testing at levels known to be suprathreshold, a no-response average should be documented by ruling out equipment errors such as improper input to the preamplifier or operator failure to activate the earphone.

Normal subject responses under the suggested test conditions should provide a highly retestable latency if a somewhat variable amplitude. Using latency data from other laboratories is not advisable because of the variation in available stimuli, preamplifier, and filter characteristics, among other factors. It is far better for the clinician to acquire his or her own normative values. Absolute range of latency in response to suprathreshold high-frequency signals is low, so that a small group of normal responses will provide a basis for determining the latency range. Once normal responses can be easily identified and repeated, data interpretation can be attempted.

Once patient state is adequate for testing, the variables should be selected to elicit a response that is as easily detected as possible. With these general considerations, the procedure for site-of-lesion testing becomes a checklist.

1. *Appropriate intensity.* Increase intensity to increase detectability of waves.
2. *Set repetition rate.* Increase to eliminate or decrease all but wave V, but decrease to enhance earlier waves.
3. *Determine size of sample.* Increase to eliminate noise; decrease if time is a consideration.
4. *Set dwell time.* Ten milliseconds is sufficient for normal adults but a 20 msec sweep time may be necessary to see brainstem responses in young patients and in abnormal brainstems.
5. *Vary amplitude amplification.* Set amplification of the baseline as high as possible without saturating the preamplifier.
6. *Set preamplifier filters to the best compromise of elimination of noise without clipping the response.* For many commercial systems 3000 Hz is the upper end of the clinically useful frequencies, whereas 20

to 150 Hz may be selected as the low pass, depending on equipment, external noise, and desired response characteristics.

7. *Choose ear to be stimulated.* Begin with better ear, if known. Binaural testing should also be considered because it can save time in some situations and provide significant findings in site-of-lesion analysis in others.

8. *Set artifact rejection rate for reasonable response acquisition.* This is determined by the nature of the rejection system in the equipment.

Once the variables are appropriately selected, the clinician is ready to obtain the auditory brainstem responses.

TROUBLESHOOTING

The following outline includes some of the problems encountered clinically in ABR measurement. It is by no means exhaustive, but includes common problems that can be anticipated in clinical settings.

1. A major source of recording error is at the connection of the electrode to the patient. If the average is noisy, recheck the electrode resistance. Resistances may vary during testing, particularly with paste-and-tape as opposed to collodion application. Rebalancing them to less than 5000 ohms will reduce noise. If background noise is not reduced after reapplication, the electrodes should be tested for failure or simply replaced, since the problem may be on the electrode connector to the preamplifier.

2. Occasionally electrode-to-skin contact will be adequate, but there will be an electrical transmission barrier, for example, a steel prosthesis or some type of indwelling shunt. Patient history or prior radiologic data will allow the clinician to identify such contaminants. Electrode placement must be varied; in some cases even recording with the contralateral side as the reference site is a possibility if the clinician is careful to interpret the response with this bias in mind.

3. Large artifacts may represent implants such as a pacemaker. (In such cases extra care to ground the patient is important.) Because these artifacts are large and not time-locked to the stimulus, it may be possible to acquire a response by eliminating artifact reject. A small sample, for instance 512 stimuli, may contain less artifact bias than the normal run. If such averages yield unusual responses, it is not possible to make a valid interpretation. The artifact must be eliminated. If this is not possible, the procedure should be terminated in favor of other techniques.

4. Electrical line noise is a common artifact. The test setting should provide a common ground and a proper grounding connection with care to eliminate ground loops. Experimenting with different power plugs within reach may uncover a quieter line, isolated from other electrical noise. Although routine administration should provide shielding against chronic

electrical interference, it is not so straightforward in the operating room or intensive care unit. Sampling different power outlets with a grounded connection in the area may produce an isolated power source.

Excessive 60 Hz noise may also reflect an unused input not shorted to ground or an "open" electrode. Making sure that the preamplifier connectors are properly in line and that the electrodes are in good contact will eliminate one source. Straightening power cables and electrode wires will eliminate another cause of such noise. Unplugging unnecessary equipment may also remove error. Fluorescent lights should be turned off, since they are often a noise source.

5.   Radiofrequency noise can create a large artifact and is sometimes difficult to eliminate. Trial-and-error repositioning of the equipment and the patient will generally lower this artifact level to adequate quiet. Raising the low-frequency preamplifier cut may also help. In some situations cable and room shielding are necessary.

6.   Unrepeatable wave forms can cause a false impression of abnormality. Before the clinician blames an abnormal or absent response on the patient's auditory response, technical errors (including electrode failure as described earlier) should be considered.

  a. Although timer failure is not common, it is possible for the timer to become asynchronous, so that stimuli will be heard in cadence or code. Depending on the nature of the failure, the result can provide bizarre and unrepeatable responses. The patient or the clinician can often detect this problem by listening for cadence or beats.

  b. Verify acoustic stimulation to the ear under test by listening to the earphones to rule out equipment failure or improper procedure choice.

  c. Recheck electrode resistance.

  d. Attempt repetition of the pattern; the confirmation of abnormality is its reproducibility. It should be noted that some lesions are not static and will not be subject to retest.

  e. Sound intensity should be varied to determine whether the abnormal responses are in fact auditory in origin. Both amplitude and latency should change with variation in intensity. If the abnormality is gross enough to make it difficult to identify and label the auditory responses, increasing the repetition rate significantly should diminish all other auditory responses, and the persisting bump can be suspected as wave V.

  f. Repeat the average with a silent run but with all other variables held constant. If the response was auditory in origin it will disappear. Anything remaining is an equipment or ground problem, typically 60 Hz noise.

  g. Consider potential patient artifacts from major problems such as noisy EEG (obscuring acoustic responses) to such problems as collapsing canals or other conduction impairment reducing signal intensity to the inner ear.

h. If an abnormality—especially no response—persists, the examiner should immediately retest a known normal subject under the same conditions to prove the equipment. (This check, if successful, may be followed by patient retest.) This alternative is sometimes the only accessible double check and is important even if somewhat time consuming.

If the response is variable on retest, a quiet run is virtually straight, and other artifacts have been eliminated, the nature of the lesion can be assumed to be a factor. The clinician can help document patient variability by repeating the procedure with the subject under sedation to rule out myogenic or other patient artifact. It is clinically useful information to demonstrate patient response variation.

In summary, troubleshooting should include a methodical check on manipulation of the instrumentation and proper patient management. Regular recalibration and periodic monitoring of a known normal subject and a daily check of earphone voluntary threshold should be routine and are as important as standard "biological calibration of the audiometer."

REFERENCES

1. Davis, H.: Principles of electric response audiometry. Ann Otol Rhinol Laryngol 85 (Suppl 28):1–96, 1976.
2. Skinner, P. H.: Electroencephalic response audiometry. *In* Katz, J. (ed.): *Handbook of Clinical Audiology,* 2nd ed., pp. 311–327. Baltimore, Williams & Wilkins Co., 1978.
3. Jewett, D. L., Romano, M. N., and Williston, J. S.: Human auditory evoked potentials: Possible brainstem components detected on the scalp. Science 167:1517–1518, 1970.
4. Coats, A., and Martin, J.: Human auditory nerve action potentials and brainstem evoked responses: Effects of audiogram shape and lesion location. Arch Otolaryngol 103:605–623, 1977.
5. Jerger, J., Mauldin, L., and Anthony, L.: Brain-stem evoked response audiometry. Audiol Hear Educ 4:17, 1978.
6. Selters, W. A., and Brackmann, D. E.: Acoustic tumor detection with brainstem electric response audiometry. Arch Otolaryngol 103:181–187, 1977.
7. Beattie, R. C., and Boyd, R.: Effects of click duration on the latency of the early evoked response. J Speech Hear Res 27:70–76, 1984.
8. Mokotoff, B., Schulmann-Galambos, C., and Galambos, R.: Brainstem auditory evoked responses in children. Arch Otolaryngol 103:38–43, 1977.
9. Stockard, J. J., and Rossiter, V. S.: Clinical and pathologic correlates of brainstem auditory response abnormalities. Neurology 27:316–325, 1977.
10. Starr, A., and Hamilton, A. F.: Correlation between confirmed sites of neurological lesions and abnormalities of far-field auditory brainstem response. Electroencephalogr Clin Neurophysiol 41:595–608, 1976.
11. Clemis, J. D., and McGee, T.: Brainstem electric response audiometry in the differential diagnosis of acoustic tumors. Laryngoscope 89:31–42, 1979.
12. Glasscock, M. E., Jackson, C. G., Josey, A. F., Dickens, J. R. E., and

Wiet, R.: Brainstem evoked response audiometry in a clinical practice. Laryngoscope 89:1021–1035, 1979.

13. Goff, W. R., Williamson, P. D., van Gilder, J. C., et al.: Neural origins of long latency evoked potentials recorded from the depth and cortical surface of the brain in man. Brussels, Proceedings of the International Symposium on Cerebral Evoked Potentials in Man, 1979.

14. Morgan, S. N., Mackey-Hargadine, J., Aguilar, E. A., and Jahrsdoerfer, R. A.: Neuro-otologic applications of simultaneous multi-channel auditory evoked response recordings. Laryng 94:883–889, 1984.

15. Berlin, C. I., and Dobie, R. A.: Electrophysiological measures of auditory function via electrocochleography and brainstem evoked response. *In* Rintelmann, W. F. (ed.): *Hearing Assessment.* Baltimore, University Park Press, 1979.

16. Starr, A., and Achor J.: Auditory brainstem response in neurological disease. Arch Neurol 32:761–768, 1975.

17. Stockard, J. J., and Jones, T. A.: Central nervous system drugs and the brainstem evoked response. Electroencephalogr Clin Neurophysiol 43:550, 1977.

18. Squires, K. C., Chu, N., and Starr, A.: Acute effects of alcohol on auditory brainstem potentials in man. Science 201:174–176, 1978.

19. Fria, T. J., and Sabo, D. L.: The use of brainstem auditory electric responses in children: Practical considerations. Hear Aid J March:30–32, 1979.

20. Eggermont, J. J., Odenthal, D. W., Schmidt, P. H., and Spoor, A.: Electrocochleography: Basic principles and clinical applications. Acta Otolaryngol 316:1–84, 1979.

21. Weber, B. A., and Fujikawa, S. M.: Brainstem evoked response (BER) audiometry at various stimulus presentation rates. J Am Audiol Soc 3:59, 1977.

22. Thornton, A. R. D., and Coleman, M. J.: The adaptation of cochlear and brainstem auditory evoked potentials in humans. Electroencephalogr Clin Neurophysiol 39:399–406, 1975.

23. Daly, D. R., Rosen, T. T., Aung, M. U., and Daly D. D.: Early evoked potential in patients with acoustic neuroma. Electroencephalogr Clin Neurophysiol 43:151–159, 1977.

24. Josey, A. F.: Clinical applications of auditory brainstem response in site of lesion testing. *In* Katz, J. (ed.): *Handbook of Clinical Audiology,* 2nd ed.

25. Gerling, I. J., and Finitzo-Hieber, T.: Auditory brainstem response with high stimulus rates in normal and patient populations. Ann Otol Rhinol Laryngol 92:119–123, 1983.

26. Sanders, J. W., Josey, A. F., and Glasscock, M.: Audiologic evaluation in cochlear and eighth nerve disorders. Arch Otolaryngol 100:283–289, 1974.

27. Hayes, D.: Effect of degree of hearing loss on diagnostic audiometric tests. Am J Otology 2:91–96, 1980.

28. Sanders, J. W., Schwartz, D. M., and Handelsman, J. H.: Effect of audiometric contour on the auditory brainstem response. Paper presented at the Convention of the American Speech-Language and Hearing Assoc., San Francisco, 1984.

29. Schwartz, D., and Berry, G.: Normative aspects of the ABR. *In* Jacobson, J. T. (ed.): *The Auditory Brainstem Response.* San Diego, College Hill Press Inc., 1985.

30. Stockard, J. J., Stockard, J. G., and Sharbrough, F. W.: Nonpathological factors influencing brainstem auditory evoked potentials. Am J EEG Technol 18:177–209, 1978.

31. Jerger, J., and Hall, J.: Effects of age and sex on the auditory brainstem response. Archives of Otolaryngology 106:382–391, 1980.
32. Hecox, K., and Galambos, R.: Brainstem auditory evoked responses in human infants and adults. Arch Otolaryngol 99:30–33, 1974.
33. Musiek, F., Kibbe, K., Rackliffe, L., and Weider, D.: The auditory brainstem response I–V amplitude ratio in normal, cochlear and retrocochlear ears. Ear and Hearing 5:52–55, 1984.

CHAPTER FOUR

CLINICAL APPLICATIONS
OF ABR

Auditory evoked potentials were identified in the human electroencephalogram (EEG) by Davis in 1939.[1] The application of biological averaging concepts and the development of averaging computer technology in 1961 have propelled this laboratory technique into the mainstream of clinical audiology and neurotology. As equipment is updated and experience is expanded, specialized areas of application continue to be proposed. It is the clinical usefulness of this technique to which this chapter is directed.

BASIC INFORMATION

Myriad auditory electric responses have been described and monitored at varying latencies from their stimulated initiation. Responses are generally grouped, based on their individual latencies, into (1) slow, cortical responses—50 to 60 msec, (2) middle responses—12 to 50 msec, and (3) fast responses—occurring within the first 10 msec. It is the fast responses, including those from the cochlear and brainstem pathways, that are clinically the most useful and that comprise the measured activity of auditory brainstem responses (ABR).

Auditory electric brainstem responses represent far-field reflections of electrical events occurring within the auditory pathway from the cochlear end-organ as they proceed through brainstem pathways to the auditory cortex. Since electrodes are not in direct contact with the neurophysiologic electric generators themselves, "far field" recording is necessary. By convention,[2,3] the recording is represented by a series of waves, each identified by a Roman numeral. Wave I has been accepted as representing the eighth-nerve action potential. All subsequent waves, however, must realistically be assumed to represent the combined electrical input of multiple contributory centers throughout the auditory pathway. Several investigators have suggested that each wave may be the product of a specific neural generator.[4-7] In this scheme, wave II is thought to be generated by the cochlear nuclei, wave III by the superior olivary complex, wave IV within the lateral lemniscus, and wave V by the inferior colliculus. Waves VI and VII represent unknown centers, as suggested by Starr and Achor.[14] Although this interpretation has its useful aspects, it is an oversimplification and can cause confusion in the interpretation of the patient response. With intraoperative recordings, Møller and colleagues[8] have demonstrated that waves I and II both reflect eighth nerve activity; wave III represents a response mediated at the level of the cochlear nucleus. Wave IV represents third-order neurons, mostly those located in the superior olivary complex and to some extent those third-order neurons in the cochlear nucleus and the nucleus of the lateral lemniscus. Wave V is predominantly representative of function at the level of the lateral lemniscus. These correlations differ from those obtained with direct recordings in experimental animals but are consistent with intraoperative data with the more complicated anatomic structure found in humans.[9]

Whatever the anatomic origin of the response, wave V has been established as the most stable and is the most clinically useful. Wave V latency and its relation to other waveforms and to the stimulus compose the primary data evaluated by ABR. A more detailed analysis of the neurophysiologic and bioacoustic principles of recording as they relate to the generation and interpretation of data can be found in Chapter 3.

Wave V latency and the ABR audiogram are determined by stimulus parameters, cochlear function, and neural transmission along both the eighth nerve and the brainstem auditory pathways.[10] The response is objective, with variations in states of arousal, awareness, or attention being irrelevant. This is, then, an objective method for the direct evaluation of auditory function from the cochlear end-organ up to and including the auditory centers of the brainstem. The ability to localize auditory pathology to the cochlea, the eight nerve, or the central transmission pathways remarkably expands the cochlear versus retrocochlear behavioral limitation. Each anatomic contributor to the auditory response can be considered separately, giving "site-of-lesion" testing its purest definition.

Site-of-lesion determination can be expanded indirectly to include those forms of pathologic processes that impose functional abnormalities in auditory function as an extrinsic force or perhaps as a more diffuse process. Specifically, lesions of the cerebellopontine angle, the eight nerve, or the temporal bone often will produce effects altering normal auditory function. Objective documentation of brainstem pathology in the form of demyelinating disease, neoplasia, or vascular embarrassment can be made as a result of their effects on brainstem auditory pathways.

In addition to the classic site-of-lesion testing so applicable to the clinical practice of neurotology,[11–13] the utility of ABR to site-of-lesion determination within the field of neurology has been established.[5,14] ABR is also an objective evaluator of auditory function in the assessment of peripheral threshold sensitivity.[15–17] Being more sensitive and objective in the evaluation of site-of-lesion and peripheral system functional integrity, ABR emerges a repeatable and reliable reinforcement of standard behavioral audiology protocols.

ABR neither replaces the standard site-of-lesion formats nor does it render behavioral audiometry obsolete. Rather, it serves an adjunctive role as an integral part of the diagnostic plan individually formulated to evaluate the complaint of the neurotologic patient.

NEUROTOLOGIC EVALUATION

When ABR is used as part of a neurotologic evaluation site-of-lesion determination, differentiating cochlear from retrocochlear disease (including acoustic tumor) is its most crucial diagnostic function. The presence or absence of wave V, its latency, and an analysis of central conduction times are the most vital determinants.

The neurotologic test battery includes pure tone and speech audiometry, stapedial reflex decay and latency, electronystagmography (ENG), petrous pyramid X-rays, and, when indicated, ABR. An increase in diagnostic concern prompted by abnormality in any test in this battery prescribes, as necessary, the application of computed (axial) tomography (CT) scanning, with and without contract enhancement, and possibly posterior fossa myelography. A positive CT scan precludes air or contrast myelography. CT scanning is a regular part of the routine evaluation of those patients suspected of having retrocochlear disease. Lesions smaller than 1.5 cm may escape detection due to the resolving capacity of the CT scanner. To identify the small tumors, additional CT scans with air contrast or posterior fossa myelography may be indicated even if the normally enhanced CT scan is negative. This additional study is necessary if suspicion of retrocochlear pathology has been raised during other testing.

ABR is 98 percent accurate in determining surgically confirmed eighth nerve lesions.[18] Consequently, when the neurotologic evaluation, including ABR and CT scan, does not suggest retrocochlear pathology, myelography is generally deferred. Identification of significant vestibular paresis, erosion of an internal auditory canal, or other audiometric inconsistency, despite no abnormality of ABR, mandates air or contrast myelography.

As is the case with any test, the clinical utility of ABR is not without limitations. To generate the data of ABR, the stimulus must be presented at levels approximately 50 dB sound level (SL) (40 to 50 dB above threshold). The average of 1000 and 4000 Hz serves as a rule of thumb. If the average is poorer than 75 dB, as may be associated with an acoustic nerve tumor, the loss will exceed the capability of the test and will generate the concept of an "untestable ear." Similarly, retrocochlear lesions other than neurolemmoma seem to generate a higher incidence of "false negative" information than do acoustic tumors when tested using ABR.[1] Thus, there are two major limitations to proposing ABR as the single, definitive site-of-lesion determination. Rather than displace conventional site-of-lesion protocols, ABR must assume its proper perspective as a powerful adjunct to the neurotologic evaluation.

In addition to its more substantial contribution to site-of-lesion accuracy, ABR is an effective and objective evaluator of the status of the brainstem. In more specific circumstances, ABR similarly reinforces behavioral techniques in threshold testing. A more detailed description of applicability in these clinical situations follows.

CLINICAL SITUATIONS

Threshold Testing

Problems associated with assessing auditory function in difficult-to-test situations has, for years, stimulated a search for an objective indicator to complement data supplied by behavioral measures. In this regard, auditory evoked potentials have been shown to be invaluable. For threshold determination the most accurate evoked potentials are those measured by ECochG. ABR appears safer, because it requires only surface electrode placement and usually can be performed without significant anesthesia or sedation. In addition, degree of peripheral loss can be determined with a high degree of accuracy. Most investigators[7,19–23] document thresholds obtained by ABR to agree within 5 to 15 dB of those confirmed by behavioral measures in normal subjects or when lesions could be reliably assessed.

No objective neurophysiologic test analysis can replace the information obtained by standard pure tone and speech tests. These are the most reliable determinators of what a patient actually "hears." We must remember that ABR monitors only the functional integrity of the "peripheral system" up to and including the brainstem auditory centers. Cortical integrative function is not evaluated. ABR is, however, a very precise index of the efficiency with which the peripheral auditory organ receives and transmits acoustic energy. What the patient does with this acoustic information centrally can be evaluated only within standard behavioral formats.

Candidates for application of ABR to threshold determination are those cases in which behavioral techniques are not possible. Those situations in which the patient is unable or unwilling to generate a standard audiogram predominate. Infants, young children, the mentally handicapped, and malingerers compose the majority of those who are difficult to test.

There is a growing body of evidence that now confirms hearing loss as contributing to significant learning and speech disability even when these losses are mild or fluctuating. Early identification of this decreased acuity is often easier acknowledged than accomplished. With this in mind, ABR has been applied to newborn infant screening, particularly in high-risk groups.[24]

ABR in newborns and in very young children has been documented as accurate.[24-28] The facility with which ABR is applied in this situation is far superior to the practical problems of respiratory audiometry, heart rate methods, or cribogram and behavioral techniques. ABR has been particularly productive in the high-risk population of neonates admitted to intensive care units (ICUs). The use of ototoxic drugs, oxygenation abnormalities, bilirubin problems, and an otherwise high incidence of associated abnormalities justify screening of auditory function in this population. Schulman-Galambos and Galambos[24] reported an incidence of hearing loss in 2.14 percent of this high-risk group as opposed to 0 percent in a similarly tested normal population. Particularly in these high-risk groups, these researchers have recommended routine auditory screening using ABR. This screening can take place in the newborn intensive care unit if necessary. Generally the screening includes two levels, 30 to 40 dB and 60 to 70 dB, with the intention of detecting hearing impairment of even mild degrees and of highlighting those infants with potentially severe loss. It should be noted also that some of these screenings will reflect neurotologic abnormalities.

In this population, ABR is often obtained as soon as the infant is stable and review of the auditory system is medically appropriate. Although studies vary considerably, depending on such variables as pass-fail cutoff level and criteria for rating abnormality, ABR detected a significant number of hearing impairments. In studies with relatively large numbers of children, Galambos, Hicks, and Wilson[29] found a failure rate of 15.84 percent ($N = 890$); Durieux-Smith and colleagues[30] reported a failure rate of 18.8 percent ($N = 1569$); and Fria and colleagues[31] a failure rate of 13.2 percent ($N = 500$). For most studies, between 11 percent and 20 percent of the at-risk infants failed the screening. Follow-up for all the failed children was not possible, but longitudinal studies where available did reveal normal response at a later date in roughly 30 percent of these babies for a low cut-off level (30 to 40 dB).[29,31] However, for infants who also failed at the higher level, normal recordings obtained later were reported in relatively few cases.

Important to the concept of infant screening and threshold testing in the young child is the coordination of follow-up retesting and, if necessary, medical and rehabilitative management.

The several case reports with comment that follow are representative of the spectrum of the clinical applicability of ABR in threshold confirmation.

Case 1

G.F. is a 6-week-old infant girl who was the product of a complicated pregnancy. In the first trimester of the pregnancy, the mother contracted severe bilateral pyelonephritis with moderate degrees of renal failure. Sustained levels of high-dose, potentially ototoxic antibiotics were administered. Even so, disease control was poor. On several occasions, termination of the pregnancy was suggested, but the mother declined despite the significant threat posed to her own life.

At 8 months gestation, the pregnancy was terminated by the premature delivery of the 7.7 kg patient. The child's prematurity, low birthweight, hyperbilirubinemia, and exposure to high doses of potentially ototoxic antibiotics clearly placed her at high risk. Indeed we were asked to test her in a neonatal ICU.

Screening auditory tests administered in the ICU failed to demonstrate any consistent response. ABR was easily performed. Results revealed normal thresholds bilaterally and normal auditory function at least to the level of the inferior colliculus.

Comment: The ABR findings in this situation greatly relieved the child's parents who had agonized over each decision made during the mother's pregnancy. They held themselves personally responsible for even the possibility of their child's hearing loss. Continued follow-up to confirm the ABR findings and to permit evaluation of cortical integrative function will be necessary. If a hearing loss had been identified, auditory rehabilitation could have been acknowledged as a major dimension in this high-risk child's future therapeutic direction, one in which audition and language will be even more important than in normal developmental circumstances.

The diagnosis of hearing loss in young children is similarly crucial. Improved language skills and better psychosocial adjustment are the dividends of early diagnosis and hearing rehabilitation, especially in children less than 1 year of age and specifically no later than 3 years of age. ABR can be a reliable back-up to behavioral formats for this population.

Mentally and physically handicapped children constitute candidates for ABR evaluation. Inconsistent and confusing behavioral audiometric data resulting from limitations in attention span and an inability to comprehend behavioral techniques very often represent reasons for ABR testing. The objectivity and accuracy of ABR is capable of resolving problems of delayed or incompletely formulated rehabilitative treatment planning, which is often the result of inconclusive and inconsistent behavioral data.

A major problem in evaluating the accuracy of any testing technique applied to this type of situation is verification of data. Results in normal subjects[7,19–23] with behavioral follow-up confirm the accuracy of ABR; however, some question remains as to its efficiency in these very pathologic cases. Emphasis must then be appropriately placed on not any one diagnostic agent but rather a battery of tests as we do in site-of-lesion testing. Behavioral audiometry, impedance measurements, and ABR must be closely linked to responsible follow-up for data verification if and when behavioral techniques afford reliable data, that is, when the child is older. In some circumstances, ECochG may be useful, especially when considering the appropriateness of amplification devices.

Although some studies report variability of evoked potentials in children, particularly during sleep or under sedation,[25-28] follow-up data on these children assessed by ABR has resolved many of these problems. Hume and Cont,[28] in a follow-up study, found 32 of 34 patients correctly diagnosed by ABR. The principal source of error identified in their study was the use of barbiturate sedation, a problem inconsistently acknowledged. Similarly, patients who had experienced encephalitis or meningitis most commonly exhibited diagnostic error. Mokotoff and associates[32] have also shown ABR to be remarkably accurate. They showed that in a majority of cases (76.5 percent), ABR confirmed the existing clinical impression. A tribute can thereby be generated to behavioral audiometry, and the concept of test battery is reinforced. ABR then serves as a reliable reinforcement of conventional testing, but also provides additional information in localizing lesions, information that may enhance rehabilitation of these problem children.

When an error is generated by ABR, rarely is the audiologist-physician team dangerously misled.[28] The most common error generated by ABR testing is the incorrect diagnosis of a hearing loss, the consequences of which are far less serious than those associated with the false diagnosis of normal hearing in the hearing-impaired child.

Case 2

D.L. is a 3-year-old white male in whom pure tone, sound field, and impedance audiometry suggested thresholds in the 60 to 70 dB range. His mother sought medical attention for him because he was nonverbal. Hearing aids had not improved communication skills appreciably. He has had recurrent otitis media and has been hospitalized twice with pneumonia.

ABR data were recorded following insertion of ventilation tubes under general anesthesia (Fig. 4–1). On the left, waves I and II were present. Only wave I was identified on the right. Total dysynchrony and obliteration of subsequent waveforms indicated severe auditory brainstem dysfunction. Thresholds were confirmed at 60 dB bilaterally.

Comment: This child represents an unusual problem of brainstem auditory pathway pathology, the etiology of which is unknown. Amplification is of little use to him, so appropriate education and rehabilitative measures were prescribed. Wave I (compound action potential) is not always as clearly defined as it is in this child.[15] When wave I is less discernible, a battery of tests including ECochG, should be employed before therapeutic recommendations can be made. In this case, however, ECochG would add nothing to diagnosis or rehabilitative strategy.

Figure 4–1. ABR, case 2, D.L. Bilateral retrocochlear pathology, specifically brainstem dysfunction. Note wave 1 preservation. See text for description. (ABR procedural recording standards apply to this tracing as well as all subsequent recordings illustrated in this chapter: 0.1-msec click duration delivered at 40 to 60 dB SL re threshold unless otherwise indicated; repetition rate of eight per second; 50-Hz lower and 3000-Hz upper filters.

Case 3

R.K. is a 12-year-old white male who was left severely psychomentally retarded as a sequela of encephalitis following vaccination for measles in early childhood. Chronic infectious ear disease made the control of an underlying seizure disorder increasingly difficult. Chronic otitis media with cholesteatoma in the right ear indicated surgical intervention. As a result of his severe mental retardation, behavioral audiometry was impossible. The child's mother and some nurses were able to communicate with him, even if on a primitive level. In fear of compromising this level of communication, we did not want to risk surgery on an only-hearing ear. Auditory information about the left ear was crucial.

ABR was performed under sedation and results confirmed normal thresholds bilaterally. Consequently, surgery was performed safely and confidently. A much different surgical approach would have been necessary had the operated ear been, as well, an only-hearing ear.

ABR is especially useful in threshold determination in situations in which accurate behavioral evaluation of auditory sensitivity is questionable as a result of the subject's unwillingness to generate a standard audiogram. By 1954, more than 40 behavioral test formats had been described to aid in defining the true level of auditory sensitivity in uncooperative patients.[33] Classically known as malingering tests, these protocols have been remarkably effective in distinguishing organic and functional disorders. Certain test patterns as well as the psychological characteristics of these subjects often leave little doubt that a hearing loss has no organic basis.

Once the diagnosis or suspicion of functional hearing loss has been made clinically by one or more behavioral tests, definition of the patient's true level of auditory ability becomes the objective. Behavioral tests can approximate thresholds in most of these cases; however, they do not satisfactorily measure the absolute or true level of auditory acuity. ABR, as a completely objective indicator of auditory function, not only confirms the existence of a functional hearing loss but also accurately defines the inconsistent patient's auditory thresholds completely without the patient's cooperation and, specifically, despite the patient's unwillingness to generate appropriate responses. Referral for psychiatric evaluation and therapy can be made with greater equanimity with objective test information at hand. McCandless and Lentz[34] report a series of 32 cases in which the usefulness of ABR was established in the determination of thresholds in these uncooperative patients. Again, we can conclude that ABR is an important reinforcement of standard protocols in difficult-to-test situations. Inclusion into the clinician's diagnostic armamentarium is recommended.

Case 4

B.B. is a 15-year-old female who underwent an appendectomy. Enjoying an uneventful recovery and 1 day prior to her discharge (1 week postoperatively) she apparently had an adverse reaction to an intramuscular injection of pain medication and became violent, combative, and irrational. Her mother defined this as a seizure, but two observing nurses would not confirm this. Several hours later, after gaining control, the patient complained of a total (bilateral) loss of hearing. Since that time her hearing "comes and goes" and will often "fade away in the middle of a conversation." Behavioral deterioration was acknowledged by the parents.

On examination, there were no positive physical findings and audiometry demonstrated no response in the right ear. Pure tone levels of 80 to 90 dB with a 50dB speech reception threshold (SRT) and 96 percent discrimination were identified in the left ear. Stenger tests were positive and communicative skills were inconsistent with thresholds.

Concerned for her daughter's hearing problems and in the absence of a specific diagnosis, the mother was distraught and was contemplating litigation against the physician and nurse who prescribed and administered the meperidol, respectively.

Under diazepam sedation, ABR confirmed normal thresholds bilaterally. This finding obviated further time-consuming and expensive evaluation, while clearly establishing future therapeutic direction. She is at this time progressing well under psychiatric management.

Attention is being directed toward increasing the amount of information generated by ABR in hard-to-test situations. Currently available ABR equipment and techniques yield accurate estimates of frequency-specific threshold sensitivity.[1,7] Although ABR is still not able to supply information equal in scope to that generated by speech audiometry, prediction of pure tone audiogram shape using ABR would greatly expand the objective capabilities of this format. Its contribution to the clinical evaluation of auditory ability of infants and other difficult or inconsistent test subjects would also be enhanced. Implied is the importance of the pure tone audiogram to diagnosis and specifically to rehabilitation through amplification.

Don and colleagues,[35] acknowledging the problems in using ABR to predict or reconstruct audiogram shape, have recently proposed using a high-pass masking technique to analyze the function of the various frequency regions within the cochlea. Using a click stimulus, they clearly demonstrated the inadequacies of evaluating the apical regions of the cochlea responsible for low-tone contributions to auditory function. Filtered clicks,[36] tone pips, and tone bursts[37-39] similarly have been shown to exhibit serious shortcomings in estimating audiogram reconstruction.

By presenting clicks in high-pass masking noise and by varying the high-pass cut-off, the frequency-specific activity from the unmasked portion of the cochlear partition can be analyzed. Using all of the advantages of the click stimulus, specifically the synchrony it elicits and a moderately complicated protocol, frequency-specific information can be clearly generated.[35] Don and colleagues declared "a reasonably accurate reconstruction of the true tone audiogram" as a potentially practical consideration. The information generated would be of monumental importance in the auditory rehabilitation of infants, of the mentally handicapped, or of any others in whom frequency-specific information is not otherwise available.

Reconstruction of audiogram shape using ABR would nicely compliment the auditory information compiled by a plot of latency-intensity functions. Hecox and Galambos[3] and Galambos and Hecox,[40] as well as Brackmann,[7] have demonstrated the capability of latency-intensity functions in the differentiation of sensory (neural) from conductive losses. These two contributions of ABR to the auditory evaluation significantly expand the restricted capability of "threshold determination" and what it means to auditory rehabilitation.

ABR, then, presents itself as an objective and accurate determination of auditory thresholds in hard-to-test situations commonly represented as behavioral failures. Screening of neonatal and infant high-risk groups and evaluation of young children, the mentally and physically handicapped, and those functional hearing-loss patients represent important clinical applications. In any situation in which the generation of standard auditory data is inconsistent or deliberately complicated by patient inability or unwillingness to cooperate, behavioral formats can be confidently reinforced by ABR. Nonetheless, ABR is not a "hearing test" in that cortical integrative function is not evaluated. Its reliability and accuracy, however, clearly make it a practical inclusion into the clinical battery of auditory threshold tests.

Site of Lesion

A number of investigators have reported the diagnostic value of ABR in localizing lesions causing neurotologic disorders.[1,12-14] ABR is particularly useful as a diagnostic adjunct in the evaluation of neurotologic disease affecting the peripheral end-organ and its central projections up to and including the auditory brainstem pathways. Its proven reliability and retest accuracy confirm ABR's place in the neurotologic test battery.

Distinguishing cochlear versus retrocochlear pathology is the crucial concern of site-of-lesion determination. ABR allows us to further subdivide the retrocochlear apparatus to consider lesions of the eighth nerve and brainstem. In the differential diagnosis of vertigo and hearing loss, the finer determination of site of lesion, in view of the commonness of these symptoms, is quite appealing.

The differential diagnosis of vertigo is not concise. Specific diagnosis is never simple. Meniere's disease must be differentiated from other etiologies, specifically acoustic tumor, other eighth nerve lesions, and brainstem disease. When a clinical diagnosis of Meniere's disease cannot be established or retrocochlear disease is not suspected, primary brainstem pathology, either neoplasia or demyelination, must be differentiated from other forms of non-Meniere's vertigo such as vestibular neuronitis, labyrinthine ischemia, positional vertigo, or functional disturbances. This is a common clinical dilemma often encountered in the presentation of the unsteady young female. ABR has demonstrated itself as a major contributor in the diagnostic confrontation of the serious afflictions, acoustic tumor and multiple sclerosis.

In assessing unilateral sensorineural hearing loss, the clinician must again entertain the diagnosis of acoustic tumor. Shia and Sheehey,[41] in their series of 1200 cases of unilateral sudden hearing loss, reported an incidence of acoustic tumor in 0.8 percent. A review of 560 acoustic tumor patients revealed that 12.6 percent will give a history of sudden onset of hearing loss.[42] In such cases, ABR complements behavioral indices of cochlear versus retrocochlear site of lesion. Furthermore, ABR's subdivision of the retrocochlear apparatus has important implications when amplification is considered as therapy.

The accuracy of ABR in determining the presence of retrocochlear eighth nerve pathology in the form of acoustic tumor exceeded 95 percent in the series reported by Glasscock and colleagues[13] and Selters and Brackmann.[11] Compression, stretching, or imposed ischemia of the auditory nerve as a result of the mass effects of these tumors alters neural transmission. It is this alteration in eighth nerve neurophysiology that is detected by ABR. Some tests in the site-of-lesion test battery accomplish this detection better than others, but ABR emerges superior in its reliability and sensitivity (see Chapter 3). In the absence of these mass effects, early diagnosis is virtually impossible and is usually made serendipitously.

A tumor mass effect is suspected when the generated responses of ABR demonstrate dysynchrony and wave V abnormalities. Dysynchrony is reflected principally in amplitude changes as well as in latency analysis of wave V and its relationship to preceding waveforms. Prolonged wave V latency represents the most sensitive detector of eighth nerve dysfunction. Brackmann and Selters achieve an improvement in test sensitivity by comparing wave V latencies in both ears (IT$_5$).[11] IT$_5$ for most patients is 0 msec, and in no case was there more than a 0.2-msec discrepancy.

However, as further experience was accrued, these authors revised their thinking regarding their original suggestion that IT$_5$ may be a reliable indicator of tumor size.[43] Correlation of IT$_5$ with tumor size has not been as consistent as originally expected. Displacement of the brainstem by large lesions often creates abnormalities in brainstem function, particularly when analyzed in the contralateral auditory system, a possibility even when the involved ear shows no auditory responsiveness. Selters reports such "off side" abnormalities in 77 percent of 55 tumors 3 cm or larger.[43] He adds AP preservation (wave) in the absence of all other waveforms as a possible clue to the presence of a large cerebellopontine angle tumor, as detected by ABR in all of 18 such cases in which this data pattern was acknowledged. Although not definitively diagnostic, this information may often be clinically useful to the otoneurosurgeon.

ABR is the most sensitive and accurate diagnostic test for acoustic tumor. False-negative rates are low and false-positive information is uniformly less than 10 percent.[11,13] In addition, no other test protocol generates more primary or objective information relative to the status of the brainstem.

The dissection of the concept of "retrocochlear" into eighth nerve and brainstem considerations proposes ABR as effective in the diagnosis of primary brainstem disorders, insofar as they affect brainstem auditory function. Starr[14] and Nodar[44] reported the accuracy of ABR not only in the detection of brainstem lesions but also in the precise localization of the anatomic site of specific lesions within the brainstem. Abnormalities of individual waveforms can be clinically interpreted as representing pathology at the site of its anatomic correlate, so that focal lesions can be precisely localized. The diffuse demyelinization of multiple sclerosis is objectively confirmed by extensive, variable waveform dysynchrony, whereas discrete lesions generate more specific patterns. For instance, a midbrain glioma might ablate waves IV and V selectively, whereas wave I might be the only waveform in evidence in a brainstem diffusely involved by multiple sclerosis.[13,45]

When considering retrocochlear auditory dysfunction, interpretation of data can be problematic. In addition to acoustic tumor, other etiologies of eighth nerve dysfunction include metabolic effects, selective fiber depopulation, degeneration, ischemia, or any other influence that might alter neural transmission. ABR is able to accurately and sensitively define, as well as localize, auditory dysfunction to the retrocochlear apparatus. It cannot, however, relate a histopathologic diagnosis. The point to be made is that all that is "retrocochlear" in ABR testing need not represent acoustic tumor in all cases. Indeed, the highest incidence of false diagnosis is generated within the context of evaluating the possibility of acoustic tumor in the presence of nonspecific sensorineural insensitivity. In such circumstances, we have described a false-positive incidence of 9 percent,[13] while Selters[43] has suggested, combining his false-positive and tumor incidence figures, an expectation of ten false-positive cases for every tumor diagnosis made when dealing with sudden sensorineural, unilateral loss. Because no acoustic tumor could be identified in these cases, test data were labelled falsely positive. It might be more appropriate, however, in light of ABR's accuracy and sensitivity, to refer to this data as "unsubstantiated" positive as opposed to "falsely" positive. Pathology obviously exists. It is, however, not the result of acoustic tumor.

When brainstem auditory pathways are involved by neurotologic disease, wave V may be abnormally latent or totally absent with any number of variations existing in preceding waveforms. Does this data represent acoustic tumor, brainstem disease, or a primary deficit in neural transmission? ABR alone cannot be counted on to accurately answer this question. ABR simply defines the existence of a problem, confirms the magnitude of its effect on auditory function, and localizes it within the auditory pathway. The term "simply" here admittedly represents a monumental understatement, for when interpreted within the enlightened context of the remainder of the neurotologic evaluation a significant contribution has been made. For instance, absence of wave V, dilation of an internal auditory meatus, reduction of vestibular response, and a positive CT scan clearly define the problem as an eighth nerve lesion. Conversely, the absence of wave V, normal behavioral audiometric data, normal internal auditory canals, "central" balance testing values and negative posterior fossa myelography strongly suggest primary brainstem disease. With the addition of ABR to the test battery, the clinician's high index of suspicion is confirmed far earlier and more accurately than ever before.

These problems must be specifically kept in mind when the unilateral sensorineural losses of Meniere's disease are subjected to diagnostic scrutiny. These losses, however, are most generally low tone in character. It is decrements in hearing confined to the higher frequencies that present ABR with its highest hurdles. Apparently cochlear lesions have little effect on latency function or central conduction time in this pathway once the phenomenon of cochlear delay has been managed by achieving adequate stimulus parameters.[13] This fact is used in defining cochlear sites of lesion and differentiating them from latency-extending retrocochlear problems. When the etiology of sensorineural hearing loss is not confirmed by standard audiometrics or when the diagnosis is not known at the onset, ABR remains accurate in determining the site of lesion, as well as confirming the degree of loss.

The necessity of incorporating ABR into an organized protocol composed of a battery of tests must be re-emphasized. The presented limitations as well as the complicated sophistication of ABR, which can subject its data to misinterpretation in the hands of the inexperienced, make it essential to retain standard indicators for mutual reinforcement.

Case 5

D.A., a 17-year-old white male, presented with no neurotologic complaint, but his family history demonstrated evidence of von Reckling-

Figure 4–2. ABR, case 5, D.A. See text for description. Absolute wave V latency on the right was 6.32 msec, clearly abnormal.

hausen's disease. He was referred for screening. His mother had bilateral eighth nerve neruolemmomas and an aunt recently underwent surgery for an acoustic tumor. The neurotologic work-up included pure tone and speech audiometry, petrous pyramid X-rays, electronystagmography (ENG), impedance audiometry with reflex testing, and CT scan. No abnormalities were detected. ABR test data revealed wave V to be absent on the left and delayed on the right (Fig. 4–2). With ABR representing the only positive test data, posterior fossa myelography was obtained. Bilateral acoustic tumors were identified. Middle fossa removal of one tumor failed to preserve hearing, whereas a similar approach to the contralateral lesion yielded excellent hearing results.

Comment: Preservation of hearing is a monumental achievement in these unfortunate patients who are often faced with the significant additional disability of diffuse neurofibromatosis within the neuraxis. This goal can be realized only through early diagnosis. ABR appears to afford, by virtue of its discrete sensitivity, the opportunity to effect early diagnosis not only in von Recklinghausen's disease, a rare entity, but also in the more common nonsyndromic acoustic neuromata. Smaller lesions define lower morbidity and mortality associated with their management. The role of ABR as a screening device in these situations is proposed. Both of this patient's siblings had normal ABRs. and similarly had no lesions on pantopaque myelography.

Case 6

M.O., a 39-year-old female, gave a 6-month history of aural fullness, fluctuant hearing, and recently, incapacitating, true, episodic vertigo associated with roaring tinnitus. All aural symptoms were left-sided.

Neurotologic examination was unremarkable. Pure-tone audiometry described a flat, sensorineural left loss of approximately 40 dB with 80 percent discrimination (Fig. 4–3). Internal auditory canal X-rays, reflex decay, modified SISI, and CT scan were all unremarkable. ENG defined

FREQUENCY IN CYCLES PER SECOND

Figure 4–3. Audiogram, case 6, M.O. See text for description. Although typical of Meniere's disease, acoustic tumor must be ruled out.

a minimally reduced left vestibular response. ABR confirmed the degree of loss and was otherwise normal. Steep latency-intensity function consistent with cochlear pathology was identified.

A diagnosis of left Meniere's disease was made and she now is being successfully managed medically.

Comment: The appropriate diagnosis was made clinically, but diagnostic exclusion of the possibility of acoustic tumor was essential. The established reliability of ABR associated with unquestioned normality of standard site-of-lesion tests in addition to no pathology on contrasted and unenhanced CT scan allowed us to confidently exclude the diagnosis of cerebellopontine angle lesion noninvasively, that is, without the need for the hospitalization, expense, and potential morbidity of posterior fossa myelography.

Case 7

M.K., a 28-year-old bricklayer, had been unable to work for 2 weeks as a result of profound unsteadiness. He did not describe true, whirling vertigo but rather a constant disequilibrium. Hearing was diminished but subjectively was stable and of no significant social concern. He volunteered no other associated neurologic symptoms.

Figure 4–4. Audiogram, case 7, M.K. See text for description.

An ataxic gait and positive Romberg test were noted on examination. Pure-tone audiometry defined bilateral, flat sensorineural hearing losses of equal magnitude of approximately 35 dB (Fig. 4–4). Speech testing showed 90 percent discrimination scores. ENG elaborated nonlocalizing findings that suggested central pathology. On ABR, wave I was identified bilaterally. total dysynchrony of all subsequent characters was noted, no wave pattern being identifiable (Fig. 4–5). A diagnosis of multiple sclerosis was suggested, although it was impossible to confirm at that time, clinically.

Comment: The sensitivity of this indicator of brainstem dysfunction is established in this case. In the ensuing 2 weeks this patient went on to exhibit slurring of his speech, internuclear opthalmoplegia, and progres-

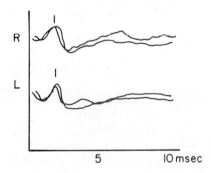

Figure 4–5. ABR, case 7, M.K. See text for description. A typical pattern representing the brainstem dysfunction of multiple sclerosis.

sive neurologic decompensation. Clinical confirmation of this dreaded diagnosis was then possible. ABR represents one of only few objective, totally noninvasive evaluations of brainstem integrity. Other currently available tests include visual evoked response and dark field adaptation studies.

fIn summary, ABR is very useful as a determinator of site of lesion in the neurotologic context. Its profound sensitivity, objectivity, and noninvasive characteristics should promote its aggressive application.

SPECIAL CIRCUMSTANCES

In addition to confirmation of thresholds and standard site-of-lesion testing, the applicability of ABR in the clinical field has expanded as equipment and techniques have been improved. The following represent variations in the application of concepts of threshold testing and site-of-lesion determination to clinical situations more rarely encountered.

Berlin and Colleagues[46] and Jerger[47] have described methods for evaluating the existence of conductive hearing loss in the hard-to-test patient. This application of ABR is based on the same principle as is the confirmation of conductive loss on the audiogram: a discrepancy between air-conducted and bone-conducted thresholds. In this setting, the click is delivered through air conduction and then bone conduction. The normative data for reference normal hearing level through the bone transducer must be established separately from that established by air conduction. The energy required to drive the oscillator and its tolerance for the signal confines the sensation level at normal to an upper limit of about 40 dB. However, in selected cases, the test may simplify the detection of air–bone gap.

Case 8

A.T., a 9-month-old boy, was found to have a severe hearing loss bilaterally. It was suspected to have occurred after an upper respiratory infection which occurred after a prolonged high fever and brief hospitalization with viral meningitis. At the time of his hospitalization, bilateral otitis media was noted. Six weeks later examination was obtained with difficulty, but infection appeared to be resolved. On behavioral audiometry, threshold was 70 dB, although the child was not consistent.

A.T. was able to sleep with his parents' encouragement so that ABR was attempted without difficulty. Threshold to click through the earphone was 75 dB nHL. Bone-conducted click threshold was 35 dB nHL, so that in one or both ears an air–bone discrepancy was present and conductive disorder presumed. Impedance audiometry revealed normal tymapon-grams bilaterally. Testing with ear level amplification behaviorally revealed high tolerance, awareness levels of 20 dB bilaterally, and marked improvement in response consistency. Further otologic management included periodic recheck and more comprehensive otologic work-up in the future. The air and bone ABR helped in confirming the presence of hearing loss and its nature so that aggressive rehabilitative management could proceed with minimal delay.

Similarly with a less cooperative child, the ABR may assist in the planning of the amplification program for a hard-to-test patient. In this instance, the signal is delivered through the sound field at a preset distance from the microphone of the hearing aid or the ear in the unaided condition. Aided responses are compared to unaided responses obtained with the earphone. Because this procedure can be done with the child sleeping, response retest reliability is high. This procedure allows for determining amount of gain needed by evaluating degree of loss present. It provides a means of detecting problems with tolerance as demonstrated by a steep latency-intensity function. Finally, the aided ABR can determine the adequacy of the amplifier under test.

Case 9

C.P., a 5-month-old boy, was suspected to have a severe hearing loss by virtue of hereditary hearing loss in the family. At 5 months of age, he was seen for behavioral testing with marked inconsistency but indication of significant loss. His otologic examination was unremarkable except for the positive family history. ABR was obtained and results indicated 50 dB thresholds bilaterally with steep latency-intensity functions in both ears. He was tested with mild gain hearing aids with custom earmolds to establish gain settings for 20 to 30 dB nHL thresholds by ABR. After several weeks' trial, speech awareness levels in the sound field were more consistent and were in general agreement with the ABR. When the child was 10 months of age, observation of his alerting to warbled tones aided and unaided remained in agreement with the degree of loss estimated from the ABR and with the recommendations for amplification.

In the field of pediatric audiology, the ABR can help to shorten the time from suspicion to confirmation to remediation.

The use of ABR in the field of neurology has been expanded to include a role in the determination of brain death. The application of electric response audiometry, however, in this context is not new. Cortical responses and EEG data were measured in 1973 by Trojaborg and Jorgenson[48] in an attempt to diagnose brain death. Inconsistent and generally unreliable data were obtained. Starr, however, has suggested ABR be included in the criteria of evaluation of brain death.[49]

In conjunction with standard clinical criteria of brain death, Starr identified in 27 patients an absent brainstem response, wave I being the only wave character inconsistently preserved.[49] In addition, he was able to follow the progressive deterioration of brainstem function in four patients who sustained acute anoxic insults. Serial brainstem audiograms demonstrated first a normal pattern followed by dissolution of the wave IV–wave V complex only to subsequently note the loss of waves II and III, and an inconsistently demonstrated abnormality in wave I. Starr, nonetheless, correctly stressed the need for ABR to be evaluated within the context of the clinical evaluation of the comatose patient. ABR is only a reflection of a single sensory function that indirectly reflects the overall integrity of the brainstem. The deaf patient, the patient with pre-existing brainstem disease, and the complexity of the test confine this objective test to an adjunctive role, complementing the patient's clinical evaluation, laboratory tests, and EEG. Auditory brainstem responses do, however, supply an objective measure of the functional status of the brainstem and in the circumstance surrounding a definition of brain death, provide data often helpful to the physician who is faced with the unenviable task of attempting to resolve this question.

In that the ABR is a monitor of brainstem function, it may be a useful tool in the evaluation of neurologic status of selected patients in coma. The rationale for the procedure is the prediction of irreversibility of the injury. For instance, the presence of normal ABR bilaterally shortly after head trauma has been found to be a prediction of good recovery even for patients in coma.[50] The improvement in short interval recordings in the first several days of the coma was a positive prognostic indicator.[51] The relative integrity of the ABR (presence of all waves) soon after the onset is also a positive sign.[51]

As equipment and experience have matured, certain technical refinements to ABR have been suggested. In addition to the traditional analysis of wave V latency in the site-of-lesion scheme of ABR, determination of central conduction time, that is, the wave III to wave V or the wave I to wave V interval, has come to be respected as a very valuable and accurate indicator of retrocochlear pathology. Coats and Martin,[52] using the concepts of inappropriate AP preservation, have proposed an interesting technical modification.

In the far-field techniques of ABR, wave I is often poorly defined, making analysis of central conduction times quite difficult if not completely impossible. Coats and Martin[52] have, therefore, suggested routine clinical use of simultaneous recording of AP and ABR responses. In this context, a dual channel recording system recording data from both the auditory meatus (or promontory) and the vertex is necessary. The simultaneous recording of eighth nerve action potentials and auditory brainstem responses, therefore, represents a technical refinement that at this time appears useful in those circumstances in which analysis of central conduction time is crucial, but in which vertex far-field techniques fail to generate the appropriate data as a result of audiogram shape or other forms of auditory pathology.

Currently, ABR can also provide data to the neurotologic surgeon during posterior cranial fossa procedures. The surgeon might wish to monitor the patient either to maintain ongoing data about the integrity of the auditory nerve or the brainstem. For instance, the patient might be undergoing a section of the vestibular division of the auditory nerve in order to eliminate otherwise uncontrollable hydrops but preserve hearing. Or the procedure might be applied to monitor eighth nerve function dur-

Figure 4–6. Serial ABR fro a patient undergoing a retrolabyrinthine nerve section. A) Prior to anesthesia during site of lesion testing. B) Patient under anesthesia prior to surgery. C) Just prior to nerve section. D) Immediately after section. E) Incision closed. F) Retest on tenth post-operative day with same conditions as A.

ing its retraction for some other neurosurgical procedure such as microvascular decompression of the seventh cranial nerve for relief of hemifacial spasm.[53] The plan is to relieve tension on the auditory nerve when changes in amplitude or latency occur and to verify auditory integrity at critical points in the procedure. The audiogram serial records in Figure 4–6 was obtained from a patient undergoing a retrolabyrinthine vestibular

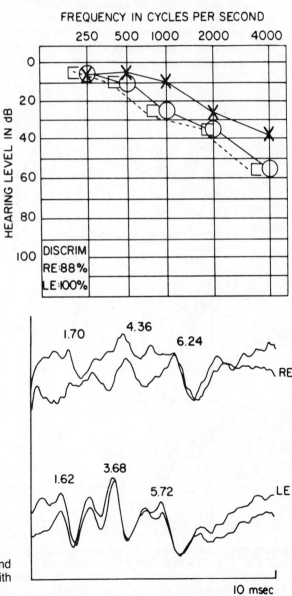

Figure 4–7. Audiogram and ABR for A.N., a patient with right acoustic nerve tumor.

nerve section. As demonstrated, no critical changes occurred even at the point of sectioning the vestibular nerve. The patient's pure tone audiogram also showed no change when retested 2 weeks postoperatively. This same procedure can be used as monitor during removal of acoustic tumors when there is an attempt to spare the auditory nerve. In this instance, the response alteration may help to predict when overheating of the nerve or adverse tension of the nerve is occurring during debulking so that a rest period of repositioning can be attempted. It also may help to determine when the auditory nerve is so traumatized that further attempts to spare it will be of little benefit; thus the tumor removal can be expedited by sectioning the involved portion of nerve as well.

Figure 4-8. Serial ABR obtained during surgery for removal of a tumor from patient A.N. A) ABR with patient under anesthesia prior to incision. B) Tumor exposed via middle fossa approach. C) Just prior to debulking. D) Tumor totally resected. E) Procedure terminated with closing of incision.

Case 10

A.N., a 47-year-old man, was referred for removal of a small (about 1 cm) acoustic tumor from the right internal auditory canal. Preoperative hearing test and ABR (Figure 4–7) indicated mild high-frequency hearing loss and prolonged wave I–wave III interval. With documentation of size

Figure 4–9.   Post-operative audiogram on A.N. at the time of discharge from hospital. Patient underwent right middle fossa acoustic tumor removal.

of the lesion in the form of a posterior fossa meylogram, the surgeon proceeded with a middle fossa approach to removal of the lesion. ABR during surgery showed no deterioration and, in fact, slight improvement at the point of the debulking (Fig. 4–8). A postoperative audiogram done on the tenth postoperative day along with ABR (Fig. 4–9) showed a slight decrease in hearing and improved ABR in comparison to a preoperative test.

By no means is the science of electric response audiometry clinically static. Experience obtained within the last 5 to 10 years with both the neurophysiologic and technical aspects of ABR foreshadows the upcoming decade as one in which a clinical explosion of information in this regard can be expected.

REFERENCES

1. Davis, H.: Principles of electric response audiometery. Ann Otol Rhinol Laryngol 85(Suppl 79):1–96, 1976.
2. Jewett, D. L., Romano, H. N., and Williston, J. S.: Human auditory evoked responses: Possible brainstem components detected on the scalp. Science 167:1517–1518, 1970.
3. Hecox, K., and Galambos, R.: Brainstem auditory evoked responses in human infants and adults. Arch Otolaryngol 99:30–33, 1974.
4. Starr, A., and Hamilton, A. E.: Correlation between confirmed sites of neurological lesions and abnormalities of far field auditory brainstem responses. Electroencephalog Clin Neurophysiol 41:595–608, 1976.
5. Stockard, J. T., and Rossiter, V. S.: Clinical and pathologic correlates of brainstem auditory response. Neurology 27:316–325, 1977.
6. Buchwald, J., and Huany, C. M.: Far field acoustic response: Origins in the CAT. Science 189:382–384, 1975.
7. Brackmann, D. E.: Electric response audiometry in a clinical practice. Laryngoscope 87(Suppl 5):1–33, 1977.
8. Møller, A. R., and Jannetta, P. J.: Neural generators of the brainstem auditory evoked potentials (BAEP). *In* Nodar, R. H., and Barber, C. (eds): *Evoked Potentials II. Second International Evoked Potentials Symposium.* Woburn, MA: Butterworth, 1984.
9. Møller, A. R., Jannetta, P. J., and Møller, M. B.: Intracranially recorded auditory nerve response in man: New interpretations of BSER. Arch Otolaryngol 108:77–82, 1982.
10. Picton, T. W., Woods, D. L., Baribeau-Braun, B. A., and Healey, T. M. G.: Evoked potential audiometery. J. Otolaryngol 6:90–118, 1977.
11. Selters, W. A., and Brackmann, D. E.: Acoustic tumor detection with brainstem electric response audiometry. Arch Otolaryngol 103:181–187, 1977.
12. Clemis, J. D., and McGee, T.: Brainstem electric response audiometery in the differential diagnosis of acoustic tumors. Laryngoscope 89:31–42, 1979.
13. Glasscock, M. E., Jackson, C. G., Josey, A. F., Dickens, J. R. E., and

Wiet, R. J.: Brainstem evoked response audiometry in clinical practice. Laryngoscope 89:1021–1034, 1979.

14. Starr, A., and Achor, L. J.: Auditory brainstem responses in neurologic disease. Arch Neurol 32:761–768, 1975.

15. Berlin, C. J., and Dobie, R. A.: Electrophysiological measures of auditory function via electrocochleograph and brainstem evoked response. *In* Rintelmann, W. F. (ed.): *Hearing Assessment*. Baltimore, University Park Press, 1979.

16. Jerger, J., Mouldin, L., and Anthony, I.: Brainstem evoked response audiometry. Audiol Hear Educ. 4:17–24, 1978.

17. Hecox, K., and Galambos, R.: Brainstem auditory evoked responses in human infants and adults. Arch Otolaryngol 99:30–33, 1974.

18. Josey, A. F., Glasscock, M. E., and Jackson, C. G. Serial auditory brainstem response evaluation in tumor patients. Presented at the American Speech-Language and Hearing Association Convention, San Francisco, November, 1984.

19. Davis, H., Hirsch, S. K., Shelnutt, J., and Bowers, C.: Further validation of evoked response audiometery (ERA). J Speech Hear Res 10:717–732, 1967.

20. McCandless, G. A., and Best, L.: Evoked responses using puretone stimuli. J Speech Hear Res 9:266–272, 1966.

21. Rapin, I., Shimmel, H., Tourk, C. M., et. al.: Evoked responses to clicks and tones of varying intensity in waking adults. Electroencephalogr Clin Neurophysiol 21:335–344, 1966.

22. Skinner, P., and Glattke, T. J.: Electrophysiologic response audiometry: State of the art. J Speech Hear Dis 62:179–198, 1977.

23. Lentz, W. E., and McCandless, G. A.: Averaged electroencephalographic audiometry in infants. J Speech Hear Dis 36:19–28, 1971.

24. Schulman-Galambos, C., and Galambos, R.: Brainstem evoked response audiometry in newborn hearing screening. Arch Otolaryngol 105:86–90, 1979.

25. Cohen, J. J., Rapin, I., Lyttle, M., and Shimmel, H.: Auditory evoked response (AER) consistency of detection in young sleeping children. Arch Otolaryngol 94:214–219, 1971.

26. Rapin, I., Schimmel, H., and Cohen, M. M.: Reliability in detecting the auditory evoked response (AER) for audiometry in sleeping subjects. Electroencephalogr Clin Neurophysiol 32:521–528, 1967.

27. Rise, D. E., Keating, L. W., Hedgecock, L. D., et. al.: A comparison of evoked response audiometery and routine clinical audiometry. Audiology 11:238–243, 1972.

28. Hume, A. L., and Cont, B. R.: Diagnosis of hearing loss in infancy by electric response audiometry. Arch Otolaryngol 103:416–418, 1977.

29. Galambos, R., Hicks, G., and Wilson, M. J.: Hearing loss in graduates of a tertiary intensive care nursery. Ear and Hearing 3:87–90, 1982.

30. Dorieux-Smith, A., Edwards, C., Hyde, M., Jacorson, J. T., Kileny, P., Picton, T., and Sanders, R.: Canadian experience in neonatal hearing screening. Paper presented at the VIIth Biennial Symposium of the International Electric Response Audiometery Study Group, Ottawa, Canada, July 1983.

31. Fria, T. J., Kurmin, K., Ashoff, F., and Sinclair-Griffith, L.: Newborn screening with the auditory brainstem response. Miniseminar, American Speech-Language and Hearing Association Convention, Toronto, November, 1982.

32. Mokotoff, M. A., Schulman-Galambos, C., and Galambos, R.: Brain stem auditory evoked responses in children. Arch Otolaryngol 103:38–43, 1977.

33. Hanley, C., and Tiffary, W. R.: Auditory malingering and psychogenic deafness. Arch Otolaryngol 60:197–201, 1954.

34. McCandless, G. A., and Lentz, W.: Evoked response (EEG) audiometry in non-organic hearing loss. Arch Otolaryngol 87:123–128, 1968.

35. Don, M., Eggermont, J. J., and Brackmann, D. E.: Reconstruction of the audiogram using brainstem responses and high pons noise masking. Ann Otol Rhinol Laryngol 88(Suppl 57): 1979.

36. Brama, I., and Sohmer, H.: Auditory nerve and brainstem responses to sound stimuli at various frequencies. Audiology 16:402–408, 1977.

37. Stillman, R. D., Monsshegian, G., and Rupert, A. L.: Early tone evoked responses in normal and hearing impaired subjects. Audiology 15:10–22, 1976.

38. Mitchell, C., and Clemis, J. D. Audiograms derived from brainstem response. Laryngoscope 87:2016–2022, 1977.

39. Davis, H., and Hirsch, S. K.: The audiometric utility of brain stem responses to low frequency sounds. Audiology 15:181–195, 1976.

40. Galambos, R., and Hecox, K.: Clinical applications of the human brainstem evoked potential to auditory stimuli. *In* Desmedt, J. E. (ed): *Progress in Clinical Neurophysiology, Vol. 2. Auditory Evoked Potentials in Man: Psychopneumocology Correlates of Evoked Potentials.* Basel, S. Karger, 1977.

41. Shia, F., and Sheehy, J.: Sudden sensorineural hearing impairment: A report of 1220 cases. Laryngoscope 86:389–398, 1976.

42. Pensak, M. L., Glasscock, M. E., Josey, A. F., Jackson, C. G., and Gulya, A. J.: Sudden hearing loss and cerebellopontine angle tumors. Laryngoscope, in press, 1985.

43. Selters, W. A., and Brackmann, D. E.: Brainstem electric response audiometery in acoustic tumor detection. *In* House, W. F., and Luetje, C. M. (eds): *Acoustic Tumors. Volume 1: Diagnosis,* pp. 225–235. Baltimore, University Park Press, 1979.

44. Nodàr, R. H., Hahn, J., and Levine, H. L.: Brainstem auditory evoked potentials in determining site of lesion of brainstem gliomas in children. Laryngoscope 90:258–265, 1980.

45. Robinson, K., and Rudge, P.: Abnormalities of the auditory evoked potentials in patients with multiple sclerosis. Brain 100:19–40, 1977.

46. Berlin, C. I., and Cullen, J. K.: Clinical experience with electrocochleography: Special applications in bone conduction. *In* Shea, J. J., and Gambaugh, G. E. (eds): *Proceedings of the Shambaugh Fifth International Workshop on Middle Ear Microsurgery and Fluctuant Hearing Loss,* pp. 68–74. Alabama, Strode Publishers, Inc., 1977.

47. Jerger, J., Mouldin, L., and Anthony, I.: Brainstem evoked response audiometry. Audiol Hear Educ 4:17–24, 1978.

48. Trojaborg, W., and Jorgenson, E. O.: Evoked cortical potentials in patients with isoelectric EEGs. Electroencephalogr Clin Neurophysiol 35:301–309, 1973.

49. Starr, A.: Auditory brainstem responses in brain death. Brain 99:543–554, 1976.

50. Argurlar, E. A., Hall, J. W., and Mackey-Hargadine, J.: Neuro-otologic evaluation of the acute severely head-injured patient: Correlations among physical findings, auditory evoked responses and computerized tomography. Paper presented at American Academy of Otolaryngology—Head and Neck Surgery, Anaheim, California, October, 1983.

51. Hecox, K. E., and Cone, B.: Prognostic importance of brainstem auditory evoked response after asphyxia. Neurology 31:1429–33, 1981.
52. Coats, A. C., and Martin, J. L.: Human auditory nerve action potentials and brainstem evoked responses. Arch Otolaryngol 103:605–622, 1977.
53. Grundy, B. L., Lina, A., Procopio, P. T., and Jannetta, P. J.: Reversible evoked potential changes with retraction of the eighth cranial nerve. Anesthesia and Analgesia 60:835–838, 1981.

CHAPTER FIVE

ABR: CLINICAL EXPERIENCE

INTRODUCTION

Auditory brainstem response (ABR) is a sensitive electrophysiologic measure of the integrity of the auditory system from end-organ through the brainstem. Clinically, the test has been firmly established to be useful in several situations (see Chapter 4), identifying both sensitively and accurately the effects of neurotologic disease on the neurophysiology of this system. Selters and Brackman,[1] Glasscock and colleagues,[2] and Josey and colleagues[3] have stressed applicability to site-of-lesion testing, the emphasis being neurotologic. Starr[4,5] and Stockard and Rossiter[6] have evaluated site of lesion from within the field of neurology. Others, notably Hecox and Galambos,[7] Jerger,[8] and Berlin,[9] have established its reliability, objectivity, and limitations in the assessment of peripheral threshold sensitivity. It was in this regard that ABR was originally incorporated into the established testing protocol designed to evaluate neurotologic disease in our practice. Over the subsequent 6 years well over 4000 patients had their neurotologic complaints evaluated by our conventional battery of tests with the addition of ABR. This chapter presents the results of this clinical experience.

METHOD

Although Chapter 3 presented a significantly more detailed demonstration of those principles and methods germane to the generation and interpretation of data by ABR, a more basic technical statement is indicated here. A summary, therefore, of our method previously described[2] is included.

The vast majority of patients included in this analysis were tested in a clinical setting, which generally afforded them a quiet, comfortable environment, ideally in a sound-treated room. The test was administered by an audiologist without physician supervision and was performed in an electrically unshielded room, the patient usually in a reclining position. The administration of adjunctive sedation or any medication, other than that which was being taken for unrelated medical problems or the pathophysiologic process under investigation, was generally not necessary. Twenty-seven adults, however, required diazepam to reduce sonomotor contaminants in the recording at some time prior to test completion. General anesthesia was used only to effect threshold testing in those infants not otherwise controllable in the test circumstance, an infrequent occurrence. Most adult patients simply fell asleep, and infants were generally tested immediately after feeding.

Gold scalp electrodes were applied, with the vertex defined as the active site and the ipsilateral mastoid as the inactive or reference site. The contralateral mastoid served as ground. Interelectrode resistances were balanced, and electrode resistance was maintained at under 5000 ohms. Modification of electrode procedures became necessary to accomodate artifacts generated from monitoring equipment, steel cranial prostheses, coronary pacemakers, and so forth.

Several signal averagers were employed over the course of data acquisition. Acoustic transients to clicks of 0.1-millisecond (msec) duration were presented through shielded TDH 39 earphones at intensities of 75 decibel hearing level (dB HL) relative to a jury of ten normal-hearing young adults. Click presentation or repetition rate was maintained at eight to 13 per second averaging 1000 to 2000 cycles per average. A dwell time, or gate, of 10 msec was employed. Responses were filtered at 50 to 150 Hz on the low end and 3000 Hz for the high end.

In addition to wave V latency, analysis of central conduction times became possible with improved definition of waves I, III, and less often VI. Amplitude changes were qualitatively evaluated. Wave V latency was compared to a mean normal 5.6 msec for women (range 5.2 to 6.4) and 5.8 for men (range 5.5 to 6.4) and was suspected to be abnormal if it exceeded the mean when stimulus characteristics achieved peak latency of wave V. This limit was extended upward for normal-hearing subjects older than age 55 years. When available, wave I latency was used to analyze central conduction time (waves I to V), the more sensitive indicator of retrocochlear pathology. In this population, normal central conduction time ranged from 3.7 to 4.4 msec with a mean of 4.0 msec. A central conduction time in excess of 4.4 msec was identified as a significant abnormality. Interaural differences were reviewed according to the criteria established by Selters and Brackmann.[8] In some cases, latency-intensity functions were plotted to provide further differentiation of site of lesion in the periphery as described by Jerger.[10] Retest latency reliability served to establish response validity. Response amplitude was qualitatively acknowledged only for marked interaural discrepancies.

CLINICAL MATERIAL

In the 6-year period from January 1977 to December 1983 we evaluated more than 4000 patients, with ABR contributing clinical information. This group represents more than 4000 cases on whom sufficient clinical data and follow-up exist to substantiate their clinical diagnoses. Histopathology is available in some cases. Excluded are those patients tested in consultation only or those who were lost to follow-up.

The character of the neurotologic practice of the Otology Group predefined site-of-lesion testing as the most common situation of applicability for ABR. However, ABR was requested in evaluating basically four clinical circumstances: (1) patients in whom initial audiologic data suggested a need for further site-of-lesion testing, (2) patients in whom standard behavioral formats failed as a result of failure or inability to cooperate or comprehend basic testing procedures, (3) malingerers or patients whose test data were inconsistent, and (4) patients in whom primary neurologic brainstem disease was suspected. For most of these cases additional audiologic, radiologic, and vestibulographic data were available for comparison with those generated by ABR.

Based on clinical diagnosis and objective substantiation, the population under study was grouped into the following categories: (1) lesions of the internal auditory canal or cerebellopontine angle, (2) Meniere's disease, (3) non-Meniere's vertigo, (4) sensorineural hearing loss, (5) primary brainstem disorders, (6) confirmation of threshold, (7) auditory processing disorders, and (8) miscellaneous (facial paralysis, otalgia, tinnitus, and so forth).

RESULTS

Group 1: Lesions of the Internal Auditory Canal or Cerebellopontine Angle

This first group was composed of 181 surgically confirmed lesions in 177 patients whose clinical situation was amenable to ABR testing. Four patients had von Recklinghausen's disease and presented bilateral acoustic neurinomata. Within this time frame an additional 23 lesions were diagnosed, all acoustic tumors, none of which was a candidate for ABR analysis. Nineteen of these 23 patients demonstrated no audiologic response above 500 Hz; the other four patients demonstrated no detectable preoperative hearing. All 23 patients were tested for "off side" abnormalities.

The population of this group included 91 males and 86 females ranging in age from 16 to 67 years (mean 43.4 years). Histologically, 162 acoustic neurinomata were identified. Sixteen were meningiomas. The remaining three unusual lesions were defined as (1) a cholesteatoma, (2) a papilloma of the choroid plexus, and (3) an angioblastic meningioma. Of the 178 acoustic tumors, 41 were small lesions (up to 1.5 cm), 101 were tumors of medium size (1.5 to 4.0 cm) and 36 lesions were 4 cm or larger.

All patients in this group were studied to varying degrees using those diagnostic tests that compose our neurotologic battery designed to evaluate and define the nature of clinically suspected retrocochlear pathology. This diagnostic protocol includes (1) a complete neurotologic historical review and physical examination, (2) an audiologic evaluation and, when indicated, ABR, (3) plain X-rays of the internal auditory canal and again, when appropriate, unenhanced and contrasted computed (axial) tomography (CT) scanning of the head, and (4) electronystagmography (ENG). Posterior fossa myelography (PFM) was occasionally necessary to confirm small tumor diagnosis.

Audiologic data included pure tone and speech results, impedance audiometry, modified Short Increment Sensitivity Index (SISI), Olsen modification of the Carhart tone decay test, and ABR. On pure tone testing, mean pure tone average ranged from 0 dB to 80 dB with a mean of 47.3 dB. Mean speech discrimination score was 55.6 percent, representing a wide range from 0 to 100 per cent. Table 5–1 summarizes these results relative to degree of loss. Comparative analysis of the efficacy of the other audiologic tests, including ABR, in this circumstance is presented in Table 5–2.

All audiologic tests were found consistent with a diagnosis of retrocochlear pathology in only 115 cases or 62.0 percent of these surgically confirmed lesions. All tests were falsely negative (including ABR) in two patients (1.7 percent). ABR results were surgically corroborated in all 181 of these lesions.

The definitive diagnosis of cerebellopontine angle lesion was roentgenographically established in all cases by either CT scanning or posterior fossa myelography. Radiologic data are summarized in Table 5–3.

TABLE 5–1. Audiometric Findings in Patients with Acoustic Tumors (N = 181)

PTA	N	PB Range	Mean
0–25	18	56–100	84.0
26–35	10	14–100	76.0
36–45	36	12–100	54.6
46–55	52	0–90	56.8
56–65	39	0–88	48.2
66–75	22	0–64	36.6
76–88	4	0–22	12.0

TABLE 5–2. Special Test Results with Acoustic Tumor Patients (N = 181)

	SISI		TDT		IRD		ABR	
Test Result	N	%	N	%	N	%	N	%
Retrocochlear	101	68.2	112	75.7	141	78.3	178	98.3
Nonretrocochlear	47	31.8	36	24.3	40	21.7	3	1.7

SISI = Short Increment Sensitivity Index   TDT = Impedance Decay Testing   IRD = Impedance Reflex Decay   ABR = Auditory Brainstem Response

TABLE 5–3.   Radiologic Data with Acoustic Tumor Patients (N = 181)

Study	Normal	Abnormal	N
PPX	34 (22.7%)	116 (77.3%)	150
CT	36 (21.4%)	132 (78.6%)	168
PFM	0 (0%)	49 (100%)	49

PPX = Plain film X-ray
CT = Computer (axial) Tomography
PFM = Posterior Fossa Myelogram

The bias of this group toward the smaller lesion is reflected in the relatively unimpressive performance of CT scanning in this population.

ENG is a relatively nonlocalizing evaluation in the cochlear versus retrocochlear context and is, therefore, considered separately. ENG was available in 120 patients, being consistent with peripheral pathology in 72.5 percent, normal in 18.3 percent, and nonlocalizing or central in 9.2 percent.

Comment

It is readily apparent from an analysis of these data on surgically confirmed lesions of the internal auditory canal and cerebellopontine angle that ABR emerges as the most accurate audiometric test for acoustic tumor detection. The sensitivity of ABR, which is nearly as important as its accuracy, merits acknowledgment in consideration of the concept of early diagnosis.

Even in those small lesions in which hearing is normal and other special tests are unrevealing, ABR has been shown to demonstrate sufficient sensitivity to identify eighth nerve lesions with a high rate of success.[10] Table 5–4 represents a comparison of the sensitivity of the various special tests, including ABR, when considering these types of lesions.

TABLE 5–4.   Auditory Test Results with Tumor Patients Related to Degree of Loss (N = 140)

		Mod SISI		TDT		IRD		ABR	
		N = 101							
PTA	N	+ %	False − %	+ %	False − %	+ %	False − %	+ %	False − %
0–25	14	38.9	61.1	21.4	78.6	42.9	57.1	29.9	7.1
26–35	9	44.4	55.6	55.6	44.4	77.8	22.2	100.0	0.0
36–45	24	80.0	20.0	70.8	72.2	87.5	12.5	95.8	4.2
46–55	41	78.0	22.0	78.0	22.0	87.8	12.2	100.0	0.0
56–65	31	83.8	16.2	77.4	22.6	93.6	6.4	100.0	0.0
66–75	17	88.2	11.8	82.3	17.7	94.1	5.9	100.0	0.0
76–88	4	100.0	0.0	100.0	0.0	100.0	0.0	100.0	0.0

Note: Only the 140 patients who were submitted to all tests are included.

Although the accuracy of the other special tests increases with the degree of loss, ABR compares favorably with the addition of accurately detecting the presence of acoustic tumor in 18 normal hearing instances. Falsely negative data were generated in only a single case. Referred for the evaluation of unilateral tinnitus, pure tone and speech audiometery as well as all special audiometric tests were unremarkable. CT scan and ENG similarly contributed little to a diagnosis. A dilated internal auditory canal, however, was identified on plain films. Posterior fossa myelography subsequently demonstrated a 1.5 cm lesion, histologically an acoustic neurinoma. The growth characteristics of this particular lesion obviously imposed little if any dysfunction in the auditory system capable of being detected by standard modern technology. The importance of the test battery is emphasized.

It is important to consider the concept of false-negative data as it relates to histopathology. Admittedly, the false-negative incidence reported in this series is quite low and inconsistent with that reported by Selters and Brackmann.[1] The diversity of the histopathology that composed this population must be acknowledged, and it is within this subgroup of "nonacoustic" cerebellopontine angle lesions that falsely negative information is most commonly generated. Our lack of experience with these more unusual pathologic entities probably accounts for the data presented herein. Consideration of this point serves to further emphasize the necessity of maintaining a battery of tests that complement and reinforce one another.

Retrospectively analyzing a group of patients exhibiting surgically confirmed lesions introduces a bias in selecting against these cases in which ABR was otherwise misleading, generating falsely positive information. False-positive findings occur for ABR as well as for other components of the diagnostic protocol designed to evaluate site of lesion. Table 5–5 summarizes the results in this series.[2,10]

Clearly, the highest incidence of this falsely positive information occurs in the analysis of undifferentiated sensorineural hearing loss. It is, however, not unreasonable to assume that a given proportion of these losses represents neural or central auditory dysfunction and that the ABR data may well represent unsubstantiated rather than falsely positive retrocochlear localization. Nonetheless, the limits of our diagnostic technol-

TABLE 5–5.   Retrocochlear Test Results with Non-Tumor Patients

Diagnosis	Meniere's Disease	SNHL	Vertigo	Miscellaneous
N	1308	902	974	170
Test				
SISI	7.7%	9.6%	DNT	DNT
TDT	10.0%	7.7%	DNT	DNT
IRD	9.9%	19.5%	13.4%	16.5%
ABR	3.8%	12.7%	1.1%	0

SNHL = Sensorineural Hearing Loss

ogy and capabilities clearly impose this inaccuracy on us and regardless of whether we call them unsubstantiated or false, the generated data still mislead us. Such an acknowledgment requires empirical definition. Overall, the incidence of false-positive information generated by ABR in all groups is approximately 5.2 percent. This figure agrees with the 8 percent incidence reported by Selters and Brackmann.[1] The fact remains that these data for ABR compare quite favorably with those generated by other tests in the protocol.

The other limitations of electric response audiometry as applied to site-of-lesion testing and already discussed in the preceding chapter should be re-emphasized. ABR is severely limited in its application when severe or profound high-tone sensorineural losses are encountered, a circumstance not uncommon when acoustic tumor is a diagnostic possibility. The inability of ABR to define type of pathology similarly represents a relative limitation. ABR is simply unable to define the pathologic etiology of the abnormal physiology that it so sensitively and accurately is able to localize. Definition of demyelinating, degenerative, or neoplastic influence exceeds that which can reasonably be expected of ABR in site-of-lesion testing.

Keeping well in mind its limitations, ABR represents a monumental contribution to the effectiveness of the neurotologic test battery. Nonetheless, test limitations relegate ABR to an adjunctive role in this battery. The reliable performance of impedance audiometry and acoustic reflex decay suggests it be routinely applied. Similarly, tone decay and SISI tests ably reinforce ABR in these instances of high-frequency hearing losses. Radiologic substantiation of the diagnosis of acoustic tumor is essential, but equally important is the role of X-ray in supporting ABR in the identification of these "nonacoustic" lesions that may, or often may not, alter auditory physiology to a detectable degree. It must be remembered that posterior fossa myelography is still the most accurate detector of acoustic tumors. ABR, however, is firmly established as the most accurate noninvasive indicator of retrocochlear pathology, and its contribution to the test battery is obvious.

The roentgenographic data, particularly with regard to the success of CT scanning in defining this type of pathology, deserves comment. Selection of this series to evaluate success of ABR biases the data by selecting better hearing cases, which generally implies lesions smaller in size. The resolving power of CT scanning rarely exceeds definition of lesions smaller than 1.5 cm.[11] We would therefore suggest that the figure of 78 percent accuracy presented here is probably unjustifiably low. Witten and Wade, for instance, describe a false-negative incidence in their total series of 13 percent.[11] It was their expressed opinion that 90 percent of acoustic tumors larger than 1.5 cm are diagnosed by CT scan. However, tumors smaller than 1.5 cm are accurately defined with this method only 50 percent of the time.

In summary, ABR appears to be the best test for the detection of acoustic tumors and other cerebellopotine angle lesions. Its reliability, sensitivity, and accuracy are established. Its role as a screening test is proposed. An inability to define the type of pathology and the concept of the untestable ear represent limitations for ABR, so standard diagnostic formats should not be supplanted. ABR presents itself as a powerful adjunct to the neurotologic diagnosis of retrocochlear pathology and has served invaluably in the evaluation of subsequent groups of patients in which the diagnosis of acoustic tumor had to be excluded.

Group 2: Meniere's Disease

Included in the second group are those patients to whom the clinical diagnosis of Meniere's disease has been appended based on the criteria established by the American Academy of Otolaryngology.[12] Cochlear and vestibular hydrops, although rare, were included. There were 1308 patients with Meniere's disease, with a slight female predominance (739 females, 559 males). Their age range was 9 to 74 years with a mean age of 47.8 years.

Audiologically, the mean pure tone average was 33.5 dB (HTL), with a range of 3.3 to 91.5 dB HTL; the average PB score was 72.6 percent, ranging from 0 to 100 percent. Special tests results including ABR are shown in Table 5–6. Radiologic data are also presented.

In this group, 1202 ears were evaluated by ENG. Again, although nonlocalizing in regard to cochlear versus retrocochlear localization, 750 (62.4 percent) demonstrated peripheral pathology, and in 118 (9.8 percent) central pathology was suggested. No abnormality was identified in 287 (23.9 percent), and results were nonlocalizing in 47 instances (3.8 percent).

Comment

Meniere's disease is a common presenting disorder in which the differential diagnosis often includes possible retrocochlear pathology, more commonly acoustic tumor but primary brainstem disorders as well. These considerations must be excluded from the clinical picture before a therapeutic protocol can be formulated to deal effectively with the peripheral process of Meniere's disease. Occasionally such an exclusion process is

TABLE 5–6. Test Results in Patients with Meniere's Disease (N = 1308)

	SISI	TDT	IRD	ABR	CT	PPX	PFM
N	*1308*	*1308*	*1308*	*1308*	*1105*	*1215*	*71*
Normal retrocochlear apparatus suggested	92.3%	90.0%	91.1%	96.2%	98.0%	89.7%	100%
Retrocochlear pathology suggested	7.7%	10.0%	9.9%	3.8%	2.0%	10.3%	0

CT = Computed Tomography   PPX = Petrous Pyramid X-rays   PFM = Posterior Fossa Myelogram quite difficult, but ostensibly ABR has made many contributions toward the objective, noninvasive resolution of this problem. Here, also, the data represent ABR as the most accurate audiologic indicator of site of lesion in this group.

Apparently cochlear lesions have little effect on absolute latencies and central conduction times in this pathway once the phenomenon of cochlear delay imposed by the hearing loss is managed.[2] More severe hearing losses, it seems, impose limitations on the efficiency of ABR in this context. In 21 patients, ABR data had to be reported as nonlocalizing as a result of test problems created by severe hearing losses (high frequency predominantly). By definition, this information must be reported as falsely positive. If, however, these 21 are excluded as "nonlocalizing," the false-positive incidence falls to only 2.2 percent as opposed to 3.8 percent reported, which includes these patients. Three patients, nonetheless, suggested retrocochlear pathology in the presence of no more than a moderate loss. It appears then that a small percentage of Meniere's patients will present misleading data on ABR but that more severe hearing losses introduce significant problems relative to the generation of reliable data. In these few cases the severity of cochlear pathology most probably prohibits the synchrony of cochlear discharge so necessary to successful evaluation of the retrocochlear system.[2] Nonetheless, emphasis must be appropriately applied to the comparison of the data generated by ABR with that of other standard tests. ABR emerges quite favorably superior to more conventional noninvasive formats.

ABR, as outlined in the preceding chapter, has contributed, in this context, to a streamlining of the evaluation of these patients with Meniere's disease toward a noninvasive emphasis. A cochlear site-of-lesion localization on ABR taken with a normal CT scan as well as an unremarkable remainder of the neurotologic test battery confers a highly accurate exclusion of retrocochlear pathology. These data, then, justify the preclusion of posterior fossa myelography, an obviously invasive agent.

Group 3: Non-Meniere's Vertigo

Group 3 was composed of those cases in which a clinical diagnosis of Meniere's disease could not be established, but in which vertigo was a prevalent problem. Included, for example, were vestibular neuronitis, labyrinthine ischemia, benign positional vertigo, and so forth. Nine hundred seventy-four patients—542 females and 482 males—were so categorized. Their ages ranged from 13 to 74 years, with a mean of 47.8 years.

Audiologically, pure tone average was 15 dB HTL with an average speech discrimination score of 88.6 percent. The results of testing, including ABR, are summarized in Table 5–7.

ENG in 863 of these cases demonstrated a normal tracing in 28 percent, peripheral pathology in 26 percent, and results suggesting central or nonlocalizing pathology in 46 percent.

TABLE 5–7.   Test Results with Non-Meniere's Vertigo

	ABR	IRD	CT	PPX	PFM
N	974	641	724	520	16
Normal retrocochlear apparatus suggested	99.8%	98.0%	100%	82.3%	100%
Retrocochlear pathology suggested	0.2%	2.0%	0	17.7%	0

Comment

ABR was consistent in all but two cases with the remainder of the neurotologic evaluation. In this context ABR served as an important adjunct in the evaluation of retrocochlear pathology, specifically acoustic tumor or primary brainstem disease, so often questioned in this group of patients in whom peripheral vestibular pathology is not often as clearly evident as it might be in Meniere's disease.

In analyzing the two patients with unconfirmed abnormal data on ABR, both demonstrated abnormal responses at wave III or later. One patient carried a diagnosis of vertebrobasilar insufficiency and an unconfirmed diagnosis of brainstem infarction. The second subject exhibited on the right a normal wave V but on the left only wave I with a questionable wave III at 4.8 msec, a pattern suggestive of brainstem pathology. It might well be that these two "false positives" are actually truly "unsubstantiated positives" representing neurologically unconfirmed brainstem pathology diagnosable in no other way.

Group 4: Sensorineural Hearing Loss

Nine hundred two subjects composed the fourth group of patients, who presented a sensorineural hearing loss to which a diagnosis could be ascribed. They included congenital losses, those thought to be hereditary, and those losses that were ototoxic, luetic, noise-induced, or viral, such as measles (Rubella) or mumps. Presbycusis was included. Five hundred thirty-eight females and 364 males averaged 54.2 years of age (range 7 to 73 years).

Pure tone averages ranged from 8.9 to 85.0 dB, with a mean of 41.3 dB and average speech scores of 76.4 percent. No patient exhibited auditory function that could not be tested. Test results, including ABR, are summarized in Table 5–8.

Of 540 patients, ENG was normal in 5.6 percent, was nonlocalizing in 30.0 percent, was suggestive of peripheral problems in 40.9 percent, and was suspicious of central pathology in 23.5 percent.

TABLE 5–8. Test Results with Patients with Sensorineural Hearing Loss

	SISI	TDT	IRD	ABR	CT	PPX	PFM
N	*902*	*902*	*902*	*902*	*798*	*702*	*61*
Normal retrocochlear apparatus suggested	90.4%	92.3%	80.5%	87.3%	97.5%	92.4%	100%
Retrocochlear pathology suggested	9.6%	7.7%	19.5%	12.7%	2.5%	8.6%	0

Comment

When the etiology of a sensorineural hearing loss (SNHL) was not confirmed by standard audiometric techniques or when the diagnosis was not known at the outset, ABR was accurate and reliable in determining the site of lesion, in ruling out acoustic tumor, and in confirming the degree of loss. Site-of-lesion capability was invaluable, particularly to the evaluation of unilateral impairment.

Once again, however, attempting to evaluate ABR results in cases of severe to profound loss proved nonlocalizing in several circumstances. Also, once again, these nonlocalizing data were included in that group representing instances in which ABR results were misleading clinically. In actuality, however, only 81 patients (9.0 percent) demonstrated abnormal findings that were clearly inconsistent with cochlear disease. Twenty patients exhibited abnormal wave V latencies, whereas another 61 patients exhibited abnormal central conductive times. In no case was wave V absent.

When this group was originally established, we anticipated a site-of-lesion dilemma in that we expected a retrocochlear abnormality would clearly be responsible for approximately 25 percent of these cases of SNHL. The data generated were somewhat surprising. Evidently the test is unable to monitor discriminate effects of selective fiber depopulation of whatever etiology, which might well alter neural transmission to an extent to which SNHL is generated.[2] ABR, nonetheless, was accurate in determining no more than a cochlear site of lesion in 87.3 percent, a surprising outcome in terms of test sensitivity.

Group 5: Brainstem Disorders

The diversity of the fifth group, both in terms of clinical diagnosis and source of referral, demands a departure from the format in which the preceding groups have been presented. Many of these cases were referred with a clinical diagnosis for ABR testing as confirmation. No universally common diagnostic protocol exists that would be presentable in this format. Each patient's presenting picture dictated an individualized diagnostic direction.

This group consists of 72 patients. Fifty-seven cases represent neurologically confirmed diagnoses of multiple sclerosis, whereas another 26 demonstrated examples of primary brainstem pathology. The following are representative cases.

Case 1

C.C. is a 16-year-old white male, originally evaluated by Vanderbilt University Medical Center and referred to the Otology Group by the Departments of Neurosurgery and Hearing and Speech Services. Sudden transient blindness with subsequent rapidly progressive decrements in auditory discrimination and ataxia presented in his evaluation. The CT scan demonstrated a large intracranial mass in the region of the third ventricle. Pure tone and speech audiometry exhibited a moderate bilateral SNHL (Fig. 5–1). Upon presentation for ABR, the patient was lethargic, incoherent, and generally slept through the procedure. Results indicated normal formulation of wave I bilaterally, normal latency of wave III bilaterally, but a surprisingly large amplitude of wave III on the left. On the right, waves IV and V were abnormally separated and a left-sided wave V was not present (Fig. 5–2).

At surgery a large tumor was found to be extrinsically compressing the quadrigeminal plate, the anatomic localization of the interior colliculus. A clinical diagnosis of benign teratoma was later histopathologically established.

Figure 5–1. Audiogram, case 1, C.C. See text for details.

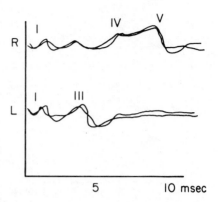

Figure 5–2. ABR, case 1, C.C. See text for description. Anatomic localization of brainstem compression is accomplished with precision. (ABR procedural recording standards apply to this tracing as well as all subsequent recordings illustrated in this chapter: 0.1-msec click duration delivered at 40 to 60 dB SL re threshold unless otherwise indicated, and slow repetition rate.

This case represents an example of the effects on brainstem auditory function by an extrinsic lesion. The resultant abnormal transmission is not only sensitively detected by ABR but also accurately localized.

Case 2

M.R., a 56-year-old female, was evaluated by Vanderbilt University Neurology Clinic with a history of multiple cerebrovascular accidents (CVA) and a number of secondary clinical deficits. Further deterioration of long-standing hearing impairment, now with right hyperacusis and tinnitus,

Figure 5–3. Audiogram, case 2, M.R. See text for description.

R

L

5   10 msec

Figure 5–4. ABR, case 2, M.R. See text for description. Wave form abnormalities and test-retest variability is characteristic of brain stem dysfunction.

prompted referral for ABR. Audiometry is shown in Figure 5–3. ABR exhibits prolongation of wave III bilaterally with poor retest on right-sided stimulation (Fig. 5–4). Two weeks post-test she suffered a fatal myocardial infarction. At necropsy, multiple brainstem hemorrhages were identified, including an infarction in the caudal pontine tegmentum. Again, ABR's refinement of the concept of site lesion is clearly illustrated.

Case 3

B.L.S., a 4-year-old male, experienced progressive clumsiness, visual disturbances, and intermittent cephalgia. Evidence of marked personality changes over a 3-day period prompted hospital admission for evaluation.

Neurologic examination was consistent with a midbrain lesion. CT scan revealed an enlarged third ventricle but no enhancing lesion. Audiometrics are shown in Figure 5–5. Acoustic reflexes were absent bilaterally with type A compliance curves; speech discrimination scores could not be obtained. ABR, obtained during sleep, elaborated repeatable but abnormal responses (Fig. 5–6). Wave I was identified bilaterally but was of unusually large amplitude. The second "bump" at the left is of unknown etiology. Binaural stimulation produced no change in wave I.

At craniotomy a large, unresectable intrinsic brainstem lesion was identified involving the anatomy up to the cochlear nuclei. A histologic diagnosis of glioma (astrocytoma) was established. The child later expired. Autopsy was not performed.

The remainder of this group was composed of 57 cases of multiple sclerosis that clinically involved brainstem pathways. All conformed to the general clinical portrait of multiple sclerosis, exhibiting clinical manifestations of multiple areas of demyelinization within the central nervous system. Symptomatic remission and exacerbation was a historical constant. Forty-one patients were referred by neurologists in an attempt to

FREQUENCY IN CYCLES PER SECOND

Figure 5–5. Audiogram, case 3, B.L.S. See text for details. Nondescript, flat, mild losses are characteristic of brainstem auditory dysfunction.

document brainstem pathology using the objectivity of ABR. Sixteen additional subjects presented for neurotologic work-up of a primary complaint of vertigo or loss of balance. As expected, a female predominance was exhibited (17 males; 40 females). Their ages ranged from 23 to 44 years (mean 33.3 years).

Audiologically pure tone thresholds were normal for all frequencies in 54 subjects. One demonstrated a mild bilateral SNHL, whereas two others had mild to moderate, but symmetric, high-frequency losses. All subjects elaborated speech discrimination scores better than 90 percent.

Figure 5–6. ABR, case 3, B.L.S. See text for description. Diffuse brainstem dysfunction is represented and multiple sclerosis is suggested. The remainder of the test battery clarified the diagnosis of tumor.

Acoustic stapedial reflexes were elicited in 53 of these patients and showed no abnormal decay characteristics. An additional three subjects when tested failed to demonstrate reflexes bilaterally in the absence of middle ear pathology. A single patient was not tested using impedance techniques.

ABR in all 57 patients showed a variety of abnormal patterns. As we might well expect in a diffuse and commonly focal demyelinating process, these abnormalities exhibited no consistent pattern. Poor response reproduction on retest as well as poor summation on binaural stimulation were frequently noted. Wave I was identified on one or both sides in 51 subjects. One of the 57 exhibited a normal wave V, this being identified only unilaterally. Figures 5–7 to 5–9 represent the range of abnormalities demonstrated by these 57 subjects.

Comment

These cases clearly illustrate that ABR can be useful in demonstrating primary or extrinsic brainstem pathology, as it reflects brainstem auditory pathway dysfunction. In the absence of any definitive, noninvasive evaluation of the status of the brainstem, both the objectivity and sensitivity of ABR herald it as a primary addition to the physician's armamentarium

Figure 5–7. ABR, A.M. This 23-year-old female has neurologically defined multiple sclerosis. Note unilateral preservation of fairly normal waveform (right).

Figure 5–8. ABR, J.N. This 32-year-old male has multiple sclerosis. ABR findings are suggestive but not "classic."

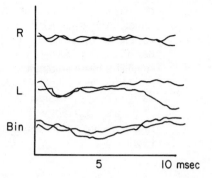

Figure 5–9. ABR, N.F. This 44-year-old female has multiple sclerosis and was very symptomatic at the time of testing. This tracing represents an extreme in waveform breakdown and dysynchrony.

available to document an often-elusive clinical diagnosis. This is particularly true when considering demyelinating processes, specifically multiple sclerosis.

The patient presenting to the otoneurosurgeon with some form of balance disturbance must clearly have multiple sclerosis added to a differential diagnosis including acoustic tumor, non-Meniere's vertigo, and so forth. In conjunction with the appropriate clinical picture, ABR findings of bilateral dysynchrony, poor test-retest reliability, and insufficient amplitude simulation on binaural stimulation all strongly suggest brainstem involvement. The capability exists not only to confirm a clinically insecure diagnosis but also to accurately localize within the brainstem neuroanatomy the "site of lesion." Starr and Achor[5] as well as Nodar[13] have clearly defined the clinical ability of ABR in this context.

Brainstem auditory responses also have been shown to vary with the stage of process of multiple sclerosis as it exists in the exacerbation–remission continuum. Possible usefulness in follow-up and perhaps in predicting exacerbation have immense therapeutic implications. These suggestions rely heavily upon the sensitivity of ABR, which is nicely exhibited in the evaluation of one of our patients who was willing to be retested once or twice a week. This female subject reported frequent episodes of the disease often achieving crisis proportions interspersed by brief periods of remission. Diagnosed years ago, she was tested 18 times over 5 months. When she reported feeling well, ABR exhibited variations from minor effects to higher levels (wave V) to complete normality, seen on only three occasions. At her clinical worst (four test occasions), no response was noted bilaterally. The intermediate 11 sessions all yielded a wave I and a wave III form. Binaural summation was only variably identified.

The abnormally large amplitudes of wave I commonly seen in these instances of brain stem pathology are also occasionally seen in the other early waveforms. This phenomenon has been observed by other clinicians,[14,15] but remains unexplained physiologically.

It is important to restate a point presented in the preceding chapter relative to the capability of ABR in establishing a diagnosis. An absent or delayed wave V does not always necessarily relate a diagnosis of acoustic tumor. Abnormal ABR data suggest a wide variety of pathologic processes, the differential diagnosis of which depends largely on the remainder of the test battery for elucidation. ABR, alone, is simply not able to suggest a histopathologic correlate to its abnormal response.

ABR, nevertheless, presents itself as possibly one of a few noninvasive objective evaluators of the status of the brainstem in the question of primary pathology. Its usefulness in the early diagnosis of an as yet neurologically unconfirmed pathology is suggested but still remains to be evaluated.

Group 6: Confirmation of Threshold

Group 6 is composed of those individuals who either could not or would not cooperate with standard audiometric formats sufficiently enough to be able to generate an audiogram. In this regard, they represented behavioral failures. Eighty-six patients (56 females and 30 males) were evaluated. They ranged in age from 2 months to 42 years, with a mean of 8.2 years. The test was positive for loss in 42 patients. None of these patients was subsequently found to have normal sensitivity. ABR overestimated the degree of loss in three young patients, suggesting moderately severe instead of moderate loss in these three patients.

For 114 patients with suspected functional loss, there was (at least) good audiologic indication of invalid threshold responses on routine testing. Poor retest reliability was most commonly encountered. In these cases otologic examination and impedance audiometry supported ABR findings. In all cases at least one audiologic evaluation was acknowledged as possibly invalid. Thirty-seven patients, after repeated attempts at behavioral testing, eventually produced repeatable data consistent with ABR thresholds. In another eight ears, ABR was found to indicate a high-frequency peripheral loss significantly better than that obtained by initial behavioral testing. In all cases, either speech reception threshold (in some speech stenger) or speech awareness thresholds were supported by the ABR thresholds.

In one infant and one severely retarded child, some objective insight into the capability of the peripheral auditory system was sought. Thresholds were obtained in approximately 1 hour, but they remain unconfirmed.

Comment

Very early in this chapter we acknowledged that the site-of-lesion surgical emphasis of the clinical practice within the Otology Group did not find confirmation of threshold to constitute a major portion of ABRs usefulness. In many otology and otolaryngology practices, particularly those in which a high percentage of the patient population is pediatric, ABR would make a more significant contribution.

Often the information generated is more specific and reliable than that obtained over a time period of two to three times longer using traditional methods. This well-established fact, nonetheless, does not preclude the contribution of these techniques, notably behavioral and impedance audiometry. ABR, one must remember, generates information regarding neurophysiologic auditory thresholds as they reflect the integrity of the peripheral mechanisms and the more central brainstem auditory projections. The technique excludes evaluation of the cortical integrative aspects that actually define "hearing" as the perception and interpretation of sound energy. This cortical integrative function is only evaluated by traditional behavioral and, by definition, subjective formats. Only speech audiometry can evaluate what a patient "hears."

Our limited experience in this category allows us to present ABR as effective reinforcement of behavioral failures. Presented as a part of a battery of tests including impedance and behavioral audiometry (and occasionally ECochG), ABR allows for an effective screening device in high-risk patients (neonates).[16] The test's objectivity defines its implied role in the therapeutic area of rehabilitation, be it psychiatric or auditory. Its acceptance as a medico-legal tool is also well established.

Group 7: Auditory Processing Disorders

Thirty children were referred for otologic evaluation of auditory processing problems or suspected learning disorders. They were unremarkable on physical examination but had frequent complaints of difficulty listening in noise, inability to follow instructions in the classroom, and inconsistent hearing. Audiograms and speech audiometry were consistent with normal sensitivity and speech discrimination ability. The neurotologic examination was otherwise unremarkable. They were referred for ABR as part of a general educational and auditory re-evaluation. Three children were found to have abnormal ABRs, confirming the suspicion of auditory problems. Further evaluation with speech and sound discrimination tests was requested to probe strengths and weaknesses in listening skills so that intervention strategies could be attempted.

Group 8: Miscellaneous

Two hundred three patients exhibited pathology not classifiable in any one of the preceding categories. Most prominent disease entities of this group included facial nerve lesions, tinnitus, relatives of patients with von Recklinghausen's disease, and glomus jugulare tumors. In addition, there was a single arteriovenous malformation, a single central nervous system disorder with unconfirmed brainstem pathology, and one case in which posterior fossa myelography was misleading. The mean age of this population was 38.2 years, with 132 female and 71 male ears represented.

Pure tone averages ranged from 0 to 42 dB with a mean of 24.2 dB. Mean PB function was 92.4 percent. Test results, including ABR, are summarized in Table 5–9.

Comment

ABR was positive in nine patients, in each of whom the study suggested brainstem pathology. One of these patients had a normal neurologic evaluation; another represented an abnormality opposite a large cholesteatoma secondary to which brainstem shift was suspected; another case exhibited a large temporoparietal arteriovenous malformation confirmed angiographically. Six of the abnormal recordings were obtained in patients with intracranial extensions of glomus jugulare lesions.

The abnormal CT scan reported was elaborated by the large cholesteatoma indirectly diagnosed as a result of its ventricle shifting effect.

A single symptomatic patient (unsteadiness) demonstrated abnormal plain petrous pyramid X-rays, and a pantopaque posterior fossa study failed to fill the suspect internal auditory canal. No filling defect or mass effect, however, was suggested. ABR and other studies were unremarkable. We suggested close follow-up and repeat studies in 6 months to 1 year. The very anxious patient, however, strongly favored the alternative of exploration. Subsequent middle fossa exposure of the internal auditory canal, preserving hearing, confirmed the normal findings suggested by ABR.

SUMMARY

Commonly referred to as "the wave of the future," ABR, based on continued clinical verification, is firmly established as "the wave of the present.[11] Its sensitivity and accuracy within its totally objective context make ABR a very practical inclusion into the neurotologist's clinical armamentarium. The expansion of the concept of "retrocochlear" into eighth nerve and brainstem confirms the utility of ABR in the site-of-lesion protocol. Its objectivity and accuracy similarly propose ABR as very effective support for behavioral and traditional format failures within the field of threshold determination. Certain limitations, however, restrict the application, in all circumstances, of this sophisticated test to operation within the context of a battery of tests, its role being entirely adjunctive.

Although remarkably useful operating within its present constraints, the future of ABR suggests unlimited utility. Increased and more detailed understanding of the neurophysiology of the auditory system, elaborated largely by ABR, suggest even greater possible contributions to the evaluation of the neurotologically impaired. An increased understanding of central auditory dysfunction and intrinsic abnormality of neural transmission alone suggest major advancements potentially created through the technology of electric response audiometry.

There is little question that ABR represents a major contribution to neurotologic diagnosis. Its incorporation into contemporary neuroaudiology is strongly suggested.

REFERENCES

1. Selters, W. A., and Brackmann, D. E.: Acoustic tumor detection with brainstem electric response audiometry. Arch Otolaryngol 103:181–187, 1977.
2. Glasscock, M. E., Jackson, C. G., Josey, A. F., Dickens, J. R. E., and Wiet, R. J.: Brainstem evoked response audiometry in a clinical practice. Laryngoscope 89:1021–1034, 1979.
3. Josey, A. F., Glasscock, M. E., and Jackson, C. G.: Abnormal brainstem auditory evoked potentials II. *In* Nodar, R. H., Barber, C. (eds.): *Evoked Potentials II,* pp. 224–228. Woburn, MA: Butterworth Publishers, 1984.
4. Starr, A., and Hamilton, A. E.: Correlation between confirmed sites of neurological lesions and abnormalities of far field auditory brainstem responses. Electroencephalogr Clin Neurophysiol 41:595–608, 1976.
5. Starr, A., and Achor, L. I.: Auditory brainstem responses in neurologic disease. Arch Neurol 32:761–768, 1975.
6. Stockard, J. T., and Rossiter, V. S.: Clinical and pathologic correlates of brainstem auditory response abnormalities. Neurology 27:316–325, 1977.
7. Hecox, K., and Galambos, R.: Brainstem auditory evoked responses in human infants and adults. Arch Otolaryngol 99:30–33, 1974.
8. Jerger, J., Mouldin, L., and Anthony, I: Brainstem evoked response audiometry. Audio-Hear Edu 4:17–24, 1978.
9. Berlin, C. I., and Dobie, R. A.: Electrophysiologic measures of auditory function via electroencephalograph and brainstem evoked response. *In* Rintelmann, W. F. (ed.): *Hearing Assessment.* Baltimore, University Park Press, 1978.
10. Josey, A. F., Jackson, C. G., and Glasscock, M. E.: Brainstem evoked response audiometry in confirmed eighth nerve tumors. Am J Otolaryngol 1:285–290, 1980.
11. Witten, R., and Wade, C. T.: Computed tomography in acoustic tumor diagnosis. *In* House, W. F., and Luetje, C. M. (eds.): *Acoustic Tumors, Vol. I: Diagnosis,* pp. 253–277. Baltimore, University Park Press, 1979.
12. Committee on Hearing and Equilibrium of the American Academy of Opthalmology and Otolaryngology. Trans Am Acad Ophthalmol Otolaryngol 76:1462, 1972.
13. Nodar, R. H., Hahn, J. Jr., and Levine, H. L.: Brainstem auditory evoked potentials in determining site of lesion of brainstem gliomas in children. Laryngoscope 90:358–265, 1980.
14. Coats, A. C., and Martin, J. L.: Human auditory nerve action potentials and brainstem evoked responses. Arch Otolaryngol 103:605–622, 1977.
15. Nodar, R. H.: Personal communication.
16. Schulman-Galambos, C., and Galambos, R.: Brainstem evoked response audiometry in newborn hearing screening. Arch Otolaryngol 105:86–90, 1979.

CHAPTER SIX

CASE STUDIES

INTRODUCTION

This chapter is an illustration of some applications of ABR. The procedure can be used to assist in determining site of lesion or as one index of auditory sensitivity and function. As Chapter 3 indicates, both protocol and interpretation vary somewhat depending on the purpose of the examination. Although the following material is by no means comprehensive, its intent is to provide case examples of the overall work-up of the patient, test interpretation, and long-term follow-up of the results. Some of the discussion will include other procedures involved in patient work-up and integration of the test data.

These illustrations are intended to highlight some questions that should be addressed before ABR can be put to best use:

1. Why is the test being done? (Is it for site of lesion? threshold data? both?)
2. What additional data (radiologic, neurologic, audiologic) are necessary for interpretation of the ABR?
3. What use will be made of the test outcome? (Will the patient be followed medically or in an audiologic or language-rehabilitation program?)

Certainly ABR is not indicated if the test does not answer a question about the presence of disease, site of lesion, or degree of loss, or if equally reliable information can be obtained by another simpler procedure without discomfort to the patient. This caveat particularly applies to threshold applications. If the patient can tell the examiner what he or she hears, the ABR provides little if any additional information. If the outcome of the test has no bearing on patient management, ABR is of use only as clinical research.

The following cases illustrate some situations in which ABR is an addition to the patient's work-up or management.

Case 1: Infant with Suspected Hearing Loss

M.C.L., an 11-month-old girl, was born at about 7 months gestation. Her birth weight was 1 pound, 6 ounces. The child was placed in the neonatal intensive care unit, and at 9 weeks she was discharged with no known developmental or physiologic problems. The mother immediately observed that the child was unresponsive to sound although she appeared alert to other stimuli. At age 8 months M.C.L. was seen by her pediatrician, who found her well developed and meeting milestones for her gestational age. The mother again remarked on the child's lack of response to sound. The pediatrician regarded the child to be at risk for hearing loss and referred the family to the local hearing and speech center. The audiologist observed the child in the sound field and concluded that her responses were immature but consistent with mild loss or less. The family requested recheck for confirmation. This time the audiologist repeated sound-field evaluation and concluded that the child was significantly impaired but that repeat testing would be required to determine the degree of impairment. Otolaryngologic evaluation was requested before further testing was attempted.

Otolaryngologic examination was unremarkable except for the history of suspected hearing loss in a significantly premature child. The

Figure 6–1. Case MCL. Sound field responses (5% warbled tones) were obtained by observation. The responses were rated as questionable, especially in the higher frequencies.

physician referred M.C.L. to a facility that specialized in evaluating young children.

On this third test, both observational responses and more objective audiologic measures were recorded and correlated. Impedance audiometery indicated reflexes present at 500 Hz bilaterally but absent at higher frequencies. Observational audiometry suggested moderate loss for low frequencies and questionable responses at 2000 and 4000 Hz (Fig. 6–1). In view of the conflict in opinion as to level of hearing in earlier tests,

Figure 6–2. MCL's ABR established threshold for click at 90 dB nHL bilaterally. No response was obtained at 80 dB nHL in either ear. Responses were obtained with the child asleep. Repetition rate was 33.1 pulses per second (pps) with filter settings 150 low cut and 3000 Hz high pass.

the otologist and audiologist agreed that ABR would provide validation and shorten the period of this initial testing.

Evaluation: At this point, the patient was seen for brainstem response evaluation. As advised, the parents shortened the nap time, and M.C.L. was tired and ready for a bottle just prior to testing. As the electrodes were applied to the forehead and ears, M.C.L.'s mother gave the bottle and cuddled her. The child slept voluntarily for the test. Responses via hand-held earphone to click (Fig. 6–2) and 1000 Hz tone pip indicated thresholds of 90 dB nHL (consistent with 75 to 80 dB voluntary threshold). At a second session with the child awake and a hearing aid selected for appropriate gain, observed responses in the sound field were improved to the mild loss level (Fig. 6–3). Unaided responses indicated severe loss but were difficult to observe consistently.

In two sessions of testing, the mother's suspicions were confirmed. The conflict in opinion was minimized by the addition of objective data. The period of decision making was significantly shortened by the overlapping test data. Finally, and most importantly, the evaluation yielded a plan for rehabilitation which could be implemented immediately.

About 2 years after this evaluation, M.C.L. has shown little change in hearing-threshold retesting, which is now obtained with play audiome-

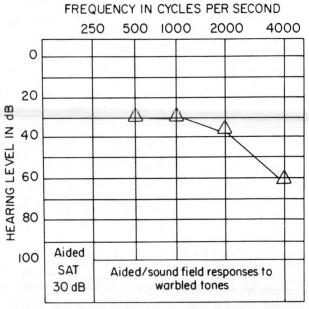

Figure 6–3. Case MCL. Aided sound field responses (5% warbled tones) were observed with considerable threshold improvement in comparison to unaided responses (Fig. 4.1) with the right ear aided.

try techniques. Her performance with binaural amplification is good and she is developing speech and language, although she continues to show more delay in this area than any other area of development.

Case 2: Adult with Suspected Auditory Nerve Tumor

C.R., a 43-year-old male, was referred for neurotologic evaluation with chief complaints of sudden hearing loss and tinnitus in the right ear occurring about 2 weeks prior to examination. During the preliminary history, C.R. denied disequilibrium or recent illness. The otologic examination was negative except for the audiologic findings of mild to moderate sensory or neural loss in the left ear with a fair speech discrimination score (Fig. 6–4). Because of the history of sudden loss, the patient was hospitalized and an evaluation was planned to rule out tumor before therapy was initiated. Radiologic screening was obtained; the plain films suggested minimal asymmetry with a large right internal auditory canal. Computerized axial tomography (CT scanning) with enhancement was negative for abnormality. Electronystagmography (ENG) showed marked decrease in left caloric response to both warm and cool stimulation. Acoustic reflexes revealed positive decay at 500 Hz but questionable response at 1000 Hz on right stimulation. ABR revealed the normal Jew-

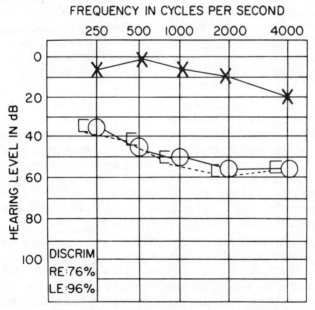

Figure 6–4. Case CR. Sudden hearing loss with mild to moderate sensory or neural loss on the right and fair speech discrimination score. See text.

Figure 6–5. Case CR. ABR results showed abnormally prolonged conduction time (2.7 msec) from Wave I to Wave III on the right. This compares with 2.1 msec for Waves I to III on the left. See text for diagnostic significance.

ett sequence on the left but a marked wave I–wave III delay on the right (Fig. 6–5). Above the level of waves I–III, the interpeak latency of waves III–V (expected to be about 2 msec) was within normal limits. The I–III shift on the right suggested the presence of retrocochlear pathology at the level of the eighth nerve or low brainstem. Because the patient history led to suspicion of acoustic tumor, the patient was admitted to the hospital for posterior fossa myelography. Results indicated a small lesion (about 1.5 cm) in the cerebellopontine angle.

An acoustic neurilemmoma was subsequently removed by the translabyrinthine approach. Although hearing was sacrificed on that side, the facial nerve was left intact at surgery with no deficit on postoperative evaluation. Deferring the evaluation would have significantly reduced the statistical probability of sparing the facial nerve as the tumor size increased.[1] As tumor size increased, it would have significantly compromised quality of life, ultimately becoming life-threatening. Short of mortality, the morbidity of the surgical procedure increases significantly when larger lesions (3.0 cm or greater) come to surgery.

Report: When reporting ABR results, the clinician should remember that the evoked potential is a study of physiology, not a static picture of anatomy. The ABR on C.R., with its marked I–III deficit, indicated a malfunction at the level of the eighth nerve or low brainstem. This malfunction could have been a vascular disorder, systemic disease, neuropathy, or any number of other problems affecting the auditory system. The history of unilateral presentation led the physician to consider the possibility of a space-occupying lesion in the cerebellopontine angle. A report of this evaluation might include the following information:

> C.R. was seen for audiologic evaluation with chief complaint of recent sudden onset of hearing loss and tinnitus in the right ear. Evaluation indicated normal hearing in the left ear but mild to moderate sensorineural hearing loss in the high frequencies in the right ear. Speech discrimination score was fair. Reflex audiometry revealed decay at 500 Hz but questionable results at 1000 Hz in the right ear. Auditory brainstem responses were obtained. Pattern was within normal limits for absolute latency and interpeak intervals on the left, but showed marked I–II–III delay on the right test with normal III–V interpeak conduction time. This response indicates retrocochlear pathology at the level of the eighth nerve on the right. If there are no other positive clinical findings, periodic retest (6 months to 1 year) is recommended.

Comment: ABR is a highly sensitive test for eighth nerve disease (see Chapter 5). Because it is sensitive for evaluating system function, it will also yield abnormal response in the presence of other significant changes or injuries to auditory response integrity. Well-integrated evaluation, including the audiogram, will determine whether the conductive and cochlear mechanisms are adequate. If the conductive disorder or the sensory loss is not known, errors in interpreting response data increase markedly. Adequate baseline testing, including routine audiologic evaluation, eliminates conductive disorders and very severe sensory losses from contaminating the results.

If ABR suggests retrocochlear response after this screening, the presence of a mass lesion must be considered, but so should metabolic, vascular, or primary neurologic disease.

Case 3: Adult with Multiple Neurologic Complaints

J.D., a 27-year-old female, presented with a month-long history of unsteadiness, reported to be incapacitating on several occasions, and severe headaches, frequent over the past year.

Evaluation. During the otologic examination, J.D. reported that 6 months ago she had experienced knife-like pain in the eyes and inability to focus for several hours, followed by fuzzy images for several days. Her neurologic and otologic history was otherwise unremarkable. She was referred for further neurotologic evaluation.

CT scan was negative. ENG suggested a central disorder. Audiologic evaluation (Fig. 6–6) was within normal limits for pure tones and speech audiometry. Visual evoked responses were abnormal. ABR results indicated bizarre responses on both right and left test (Fig. 6–7). These results suggested nonlocalized auditory brainstem abnormality. Subsequent findings in the clinical course of J.D. confirmed the presence of multiple sclerosis (MS). Repeat ABRs (Fig. 6–8) recorded the fluctuant nature of this disease.

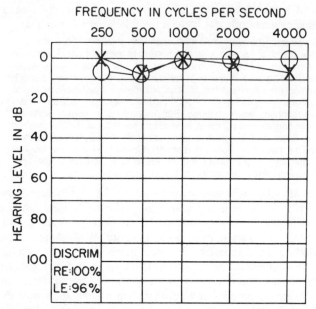

Figure 6–6. Case JD. Pure tone thresholds were within normal limits bilaterally. Speech discrimination scores were excellent in both ears. See text.

Figure 6–7. Case JD. ABR was abnormal bilaterally because only early portions of the sequence could be detected in either ear. Responses were obtained at 13.1 pps at 80 dB nHL bilaterally with standard electrode montage (see Chapter 3).

Figure 6–8. Case JD. Repeat ABR six weeks following the original study (Fig. 6.7). Results were changed in that more detail could be detected on the right, but both ears continued to be abnormal.

Comment: The presence of bilateral findings at various levels on ABR does not rule out tumor, because extra-axial lesions can yield bizarre effects. However, if there is history of nonspecific neurologic disease and MS is suspected, ABR should be considered for further evaluation of the patient. Normal response can be expected in some MS patients (23.4 percent),[2] but abnormal response can be a reflection of the presence of demyelinating disease. The abnormal finding is particularly of interest in the patient who denies auditory problems. Unstable morphology, as exhibited in this patient, is an occasional finding in this group. Abnormal threshold sensitivity with no other otologic disease is highly unusual in MS patients.

Report. ABR evaluation in such a case would be reported in the following manner.

J.D. was seen for ABR with chief complaints of loss of balance and headaches over the past several months. Preliminary audiologic evaluation indicated hearing within normal limits bilaterally and excellent speech discrimination scores. ABR was obtained (see patient record for protocol) on a well-relaxed patient and yielded abnormal patterns on both sides. On the right, wave I and wave II were identified at normal latency for a young female. Wave III was significantly delayed and the IV–V complex was abnormally small in amplitude. On the left test, waves I, II, and III were within normal limits but wave V was poorly identified. This would suggest brainstem abnormality evident on stimulation of either ear, suspected to be of diffuse or extra-axial nature. Eighth nerve disease on the right is a remote but possible second source of pathology in addition to the brainstem disease. Further audiologic or neurologic evaluation and repeat ABR should be considered.

Case 4: Adult with Sudden Hearing Loss of Unknown Etiology

J.T.L., a 27-year-old male, reported to the clinic with a report of marked decrease in hearing over 6 weeks' time. He complained of increased difficulty in hearing his wife and children at home, but even more difficulty hearing his co-workers at the plant. He had no previous history of significant otologic disease, no history of familial hearing loss, no ear disease, no noise exposure except present employment, no known exposure to ototoxic drugs, no recent illness, and no significant contributing health factors.

Evaluation: Neurologic and otologic evaluations were unremarkable except for the apparent bilateral hearing loss. CT scan of the head and routine plain X-rays of the internal auditory canals were unremarkable. ENG was negative for abnormality; laboratory data including FTA were also unremarkable. Informal evaluation revealed minimal difficulty in communication.

Audiologic test revealed poor consistency, with responses at 70 to 90 dB for pure tones and speech reception thresholds of 50 dB bilaterally (Fig. 6–9). The substantiation of suspected psychogenic hearing loss or pseudohypoacusis was initiated with acoustic reflex audiometry. When

Figure 6–9. Case JTL. Audiogram revealed discrepancy between pure tone average (500, 1000 and 2000 Hz) and speech reception threshold (SRT). Threshold retest was poor. See text.

Figure 6–10. Case JTL. ABR at 80 dB nHL at a slow rate (13.1 pps) indicated normal absolute and interpeak latencies bilaterally with I-V conduction time on the order of about 4.0 msec.

levels of reflex occurred at or below voluntary thresholds, ABR was requested. Testing at high intensity (80 dB nHL) revealed patterns with normal absolute latency values for the waves and normal interpeak latencies bilaterally (Fig. 6–10). ABR thresholds for click were obtained with responses detected as low as 20 dB in both ears (Fig. 6–11). J.T.L. was submitted to repeat routine audiologic evaluation immediately, and voluntary thresholds confirmed hearing levels within the normal to borderline loss range (Fig. 6–12).

This patient was referred for psychiatric evaluation. Further otologic and audiologic management was deferred.

Comment: ABR is an excellent tool for substantiating or disallowing a claim to hearing loss because it is considered an objective indicator. The test is abused if it is not considered in the context of the patient's report of what is heard, however, because ABR only tests synchronous discharge at the level of the cochlea and its transmission toward the cortex but not its integration at that level. Therefore, a full-scale evaluation to investigate both patient complaint and apparent audiologic discrepancies is important. Appropriate investigation may necessitate any number of tools in addition to routine audiologic evaluation, immitance testing, and ABR. Some examples are central speech tests, electrocochleography, middle latency responses, and ultra-audiometric response evaluation. Selection of the tests should be varied according to the patient presentation.

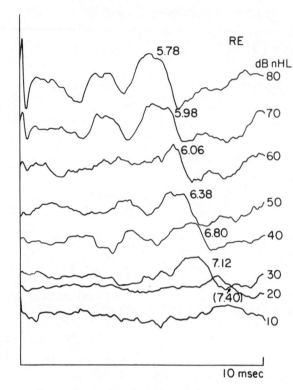

Figure 6–11. Case JTL. ABR threshold search shown for the right ear only. Threshold was 20 dB with an absolute latency of Wave V consistent with a threshold response. Left ear responses also yielded a 20 dB nHL threshold. Responses were obtained at 33.1 pps.

Report: Findings were reported as follows.

J.I.L. was seen for audiologic evaluation with the chief complaint of sudden onset of hearing loss bilaterally. Pure tone thresholds suggested severe hearing loss bilaterally but poor retest reliability with threshold range over about 20 dB. Speech reception thresholds were also variable, with better responses obtained by ascending technique than descending technique and suggesting no more than moderate loss bilaterally. Ultra-audiometric tests did not reveal exceptional high-frequency hearing and the threshold discrepancies were unresolved. Speech discrimination scores were fair when delivered at the best pure tone average bilaterally. Thresholds of the acoustic reflexes also were obtained at unacceptable levels in comparison to pure tone thresholds volunteered by the patient. Auditory brainstem responses were obtained and indicated normal retrocochlear function as reflected by this test. Thresholds were 20 dB bilaterally for click, indicating hearing (as assessed within the limited range of this procedure) to be essentially within normal limits. Retest immediately following the ABR also yielded normal threshold sensitivity across the frequency range. The patient will be re-evaluated at the request of the referring physician.

FREQUENCY IN CYCLES PER SECOND

Figure 6–12. Case JTL. Audiometry was repeated after ABR with marked improvement. SRT and PTA were in good agreement and indicated normal hearing. Speech discrimination scores at normal conversational loudness were excellent.

Case 5: Adult with Fluctuant Hearing Loss

T.K.R., a 41-year-old man, complained of fluctuant hearing loss, tinnitus, reduced noise tolerance, and pressure in the right ear. The onset, 3 years ago, was accompanied by vertigo and nausea. The episodes currently are less severe but more frequent. For the past year, hearing in the right ear no longer returned to normal between attacks. The left ear was symptom-free. Initial medical management had included diuretic and labyrinthine sedatives. When the frequency of the episodes became more aggravating, T.K.R. was referred for further evaluation to confirm the working diagnosis of Meniere's disease.

Evaluation: Otologic examination revealed no evidence of middle ear disease. There was no significant medical history to account for the disorder. Neurologic examination was unremarkable except for the report of right-ear deficit. To rule out the possibility of acoustic tumor, radiologic evaluation was initiated. Plain films were interpreted as normal but an enhanced CT scan of the head could not be obtained because of a history of allergic response to the contrast material.

At this point, the audiologic evaluation was reviewed. T.K.R. was found to have a moderately severe loss with fair speech discrimination

Figure 6–13. Case TKR. Audiogram revealed normal sensitivity on the left and moderately severe sensory or neural loss on the right. Speech discrimination scores were good on the left and fair on the right. See text.

ability on the right and normal response on the left (Fig. 6–13). Acoustic stapedial reflexes were normal on left test and occurred at reduced sensation level on the right. There was no evidence of decay. ABR was obtained.

Results indicated (1) hearing loss on the right, consistent with the audiogram (Fig. 6–14); (2) steep latency-intensity function consistent with the patient's report of loudness tolerance problems; and (3) no interpeak latency abnormality and thus no sign of retrocochlear pathology (Fig. 6–15).

Report: These findings were reported as follows:

Left ear responses were within normal limits. Right ear responses revealed threshold deficit consistent with the audiologic evaluation, cochlear abnormality in the latency-intensity function, and normal neural conduction. The impression was cochlear pathology, moderate in degree, on the right.

Comment: In view of the history of the patient, further studies were deferred. T.K.R. was submitted to a more aggressive medical regimen and advised to return in 6 months for re-evaluation. In this case, the ABR was normal and significantly lowered the index of suspicion of a retrocochlear lesion such as an acoustic nerve tumor, even though the CT scan could not be accomplished. In a case where the diagnosis is suspect, or radiologic data suggest but do not confirm an acoustic tumor, serial ABRs can assist in monitoring the lesion.

Figure 6–14. Case TKR. ABR latency intensity function on the right revealed threshold at 65 dB and steep latency-intensity function suggestive of cochlear pathology on the right. (Click rate 33.1 pps).

Routine assessment of ABR threshold is not generally indicated in a patient who cooperates for standard pure tone evaluation. In the case of suspected cochlear pathology, testing at different intensity levels may help to support the presence of inner ear disease. The finding of steep latency-

Figure 6–15. Case TKR. ABR indicated normal abrolute and interpeak latencies bilaterally (about 4.0 msec) despite the threshold differences noted on pure tone testing. Intensity was increased on the right to overcome the sensitivity loss.

intensity function appears only in cochlear pathology, although some subjects with confirmed inner ear disease do not demonstrate this.

Case 6: Patient with False-Positive ABR

K.L.C., a 57-year-old man, went to his family physician with a chief complaint of headaches, predominantly on the left side, generally in the occipital region. He reported that aspirin helped very little and at times the pain seemed to be deep in his jaw and ear. He noticed no change in hearing or difference between ears although he had acquired some loss in both ears as the result of noise exposure.

Evaluation: K.L.C.'s physician scheduled him for a CT scan of the head which was normal. ABR and visual evoked response (VER) were also obtained. VER was normal but ABR revealed delayed wave V on the left (Fig. 6–16). At this point, the physician was faced with the problem of ruling out tumor on the left by hospitalizing the patient for further radiologic evaluation or referring the patient to specialists for further evaluation of the ABR abnormality.

At a local outpatient diagnostic facility, the patient received a neurologic and otologic second opinion with no additional significant findings pending the audiologic evaluation. Hearing assessment, shown in Figure 6–17, revealed marked high-frequency loss bilaterally. The loss was more severe on the left and affected 2000 Hz as well as higher frequencies. Speech discrimination scores were fair bilaterally. Acoustic stapedial reflex decay, measured during impedance audiometry, was neg-

Figure 6–16. CASE KCL. ABR appeared normal on the right but Wave V was markedly delayed on the left. Stimulus intensity was 80 dB nHL. See text.

10 msec

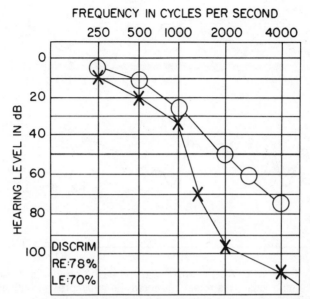

Figure 6–17. Case KCL. Thresholds showed high frequency loss bilaterally, more severe on the left. Speech discrimination scores were fair in both ears. See text.

ative bilaterally. Repeat of the ABR (Fig. 6–18) revealed normal I–V conduction time on the right but only waves III and V on the left. At increased intensity, wave V decreased in latency and was found to be within normal limits.

Report: The audiologic report indicated the asymmetry between ears but the absence of conclusive retrocochlear findings. When asked to compare the current report with previous findings, the clinician indicated that the initial test was done at inadequate intensity on the left and data could not be compared.

Comment: K.L.C. was advised of the results. The consulting physician recommended periodic re-evaluation with CT scan and auditory tests or hospitalization for posterior fossa myelogram with contrast for definitive study. Because of his anxiety about the possibility of tumor, K.L.C. elected to submit to posterior fossa myelography. The radiologist found no abnormality. Periodic otologic recheck was then initiated.

ABR can lead to significant problems with apparently abnormal results if the test is interpreted without adequate audiologic data. Because positive results necessitate consideration of significant otologic or neurologic disorder, it is important to consider every potential artifact, such as underlying hearing loss. The alternative to ignoring such factors is to submit the patient to invasive procedures such as myelography, angiography, expensive repetitive CT scans, or nuclear magnetic resonance scans.

Figure 6-18. Case KCL. ABR intensity was increased on the left to accomodate the patient's hearing loss. This retest corrected the misimpression obtained on the original ABR (Fig. 6.16) prior to obtaining the hearing test. See text.

Although the most desirable interpretative approach is baseline and cross-check auditory tests, certainly no "abnormal" ABR trace should be accepted without the underlying audiologic data.

Case 7: Seven-year-old with Audiologic Rehabilitation Failure

A.K.F., a 7½-year-old boy, had appeared to be delayed in developing speech and language skills at about 2½ years. His parents were advised at that time that hearing responses were consistent with mild loss, although probably not of sufficient magnitude to cause speech delay. At 3½ years of age, A.K.F. was re-evaluated and found to be functioning at the 24-months level on speech tasks, somewhat better for receptive language, and at 4 to 4½ years on other IQ tasks. Motor coordination skills were at age level. History (both medical and social) was negative for contributing factors. The parents reported that A.K.F. seemed to hear very well in a one-on-one situation but ignored or didn't hear otherwise.

Evaluation: At the time of the complete evaluation, A.K.F. was 3½ years old. He was referred to his family's otologist for consultation. On examination, there was no evidence of otologic disorder except for the audiogram (Fig. 6-19). The speech reception thresholds were somewhat better than expected in view of the pure tone average. Retest reliability was noted to be only fair. Speech discrimination scores were fair, poorer

Figure 6–19. Case AKF. The audiogram was described as having questionable reliability. This 3½ year old boy appeared to have mild loss for tones but normal speech reception thresholds. Pure tone retest ranged 10 to 20 dB. See text.

than expected in view of the audiogram. Polytomography and routine laboratory studies, including FTA and creatinine clearance, were negative.

A.K.F. was returned for testing with hearing aids and seemed to do somewhat better on discrimination tests. After a month's trial he began wearing a mild-gain behind-the-ear hearing aid.

At age 7½, A.K.F. returned to the otologist with his parents. They indicated that he would occasionally wear his hearing aid at home but seldom at school and that his teacher described him as behaviorally disturbed and learning delayed. The speech pathologist maintained that A.K.F. continued to make slow but steady progress. The school psychologist was leaning toward classifying A.K.F. as a behavior problem because testing placed his IQ well ahead of age level in several areas. At this time, the otologist recommended comprehensive audiologic evaluation.

Audiologic Evaluation: Audiologic tests were relatively unchanged at the time of the re-evaluation. Assessment of ultra-audiometric (frequencies above 800 Hz) response yielded moderate to severe loss so that the test discrepancies were unexplained. There was no evidence of air–bone gap. Tympanometric curves suggested normal middle ear function on both sides, but reflexes were somewhat elevated and poor in amplitude. Speech discrimination score at 60 dB hearing level in the sound field was fair but markedly reduced in the presence of cafeteria noise. Performance with amplification was no better. ABR was obtained and, as shown in Figure 6–20, the results indicated bizarre response bilaterally. Middle latency responses were also abnormal on stimulation of either ear. Unfortunately for A.K.F., results pointed to central auditory problems. This was substantiated by the child's behavior in the noisy classroom versus his performance in one-on-one testing and his failure to adjust to amplification. Indeed, the hearing aid simply decreased the signal-to-noise ratio unfavorably so that performance was probably hindered in these conditions.

Audiologic Report: The audiologist forwarded the current findings to the parents, the school system, and the otologist:

> A.K.F. was found to have a mild, mid-frequency hearing loss bilaterally with no evidence of air–bone gap. Speech reception thresholds were somewhat better than pure tone average, possibly reflecting the unusual audiometric configuration. Retest was only fair but in view of the similarity of hearing tests over several years, the validity of the hearing loss was not questioned. Speech discrimination scores were fair bilaterally.
>
> In the sound field, speech discrimination score at 60 dB HL (moderately loud conversational level) was also only fair. Increase to 70 dB HL caused minor complaints of tolerance and reduction in speech discrimination ability. At 60 dB HL in noise, aided and unaided scores were poorer than unaided score in quiet. Tympanometry yielded Type A (normal) response from both ears with elevation of reflexes bilaterally

Figure 6–20. Case AKF. ABR at high intensity (90 dB nHL) revealed markedly poor morphology in both ears suggesting eighth nerve or brainstem abnormality. The dyssynchrony ruled out latency-intensity search to obtain thresholds.

and poor amplitude, suggesting the need for further evaluation of the retrocochlear pathways.

ABR was abnormal in that few wavelets could be compared to the normal pattern though A.K.F.'s responses were highly repeatable. This finding pointed to central auditory problems. In addition, threshold assessment failed to produce responses below the 60 dB level re: normal, but these findings were held to be invalid because of the neurologic abnormalities. Middle latency responses were also abnormal, pointing again to central pathology.

Impression: Central auditory pathology suggested by history, speech audiometry and auditory evoked potentials.

Recommendations: (1) Referral for otologic re-evaluation. (2) Placement in a quiet learning environment with emphasis on visual information input as opposed to auditory emphasis. (3) Discontinuance of hearing aid use until re-assessment.

As an addendum, current trends to use assistive listening devices such as FM systems in such cases would prompt a recommendation of trial use with such a unit on A.K.F. in the classroom.

Otologic Re-evaluation: To rule out any clinically significant disease process, A.K.F. was referred for CT scan. This study, along with full neurologic evaluation, was negative. Annual recheck to update the physician on any change and to re-evaluate hearing and school performance was recommended.

Comment: Although not all listening-condition complaints, such as A.K.F.'s problems in noise, can be documented in the test situation, it is often helpful in streamlining both the evaluation and rehabilitation plan to try to replicate them. In addition, if auditory processing seems to be poor, auditory evoked potentials, including ABR, may be helpful. If, however, there is a pattern abnormality, the ability to apply the test for threshold determination will be severely limited. It is impossible to totally isolate threshold uses from site-of-lesion applications of ABR, and it is hazardous to try. Clinical findings of abnormality on the ABR warrant not only rehabilitation planning but also adequate medical assessment. Moreover, it is useless to obtain the neuroaudiologic data and then fail to follow through in the clinical and classroom management of these patients. Audiologists and language pathologists in particular have to become creative in providing individualized programs while keeping these unusual learners in the classroom.

Case 8: Adult with Family History of von Recklinghausen's Disease

R.J.T., a 21-year-old male, was referred because of family history of bilateral acoustic tumors. He had an aunt with bilateral acoustic tumors as a manifestation of von Recklinghausen's disease. Recently his sister, 2 years younger, developed sudden hearing loss in one ear and on CT scan was found to have a small (1.5 cm) tumor in that ear and a somewhat larger lesion in the opposite, normal-hearing ear. R.J.T. was referred for further evaluation.

He denied noticeable loss of hearing but did complain that his hearing was not as strong as it had been a few years before. He had occasional brief periods of high-pitched tinnitus in the left ear. He denied balance disorders or any other clinically significant otologic or neurologic symptoms. Other than childhood infections, there was no indication of prior contributing disorders. General health was excellent.

The neurotologist found the physical examination to be normal but elected to obtain further workup because of family history. He advised audiologic and radiologic evaluation.

Audiologic Evaluation: A hearing test revealed responses at the lower limits of normal hearing bilaterally (Fig. 6–21). Speech discrimination scores were excellent at normal sensation level. At high intensity, however, left-ear scores dropped significantly; right-ear responses remained intact. Acoustic stapedial reflexes were elevated bilaterally. ABR exhibited marked delay in wave V latency on the right test and delayed I–III conduction time on the left with normal conduction time between waves III and V (Fig. 6–22). An increased intensity series did not improve the

Figure 6–21. Case RJT. Audiogram indicated hearing at the lower limits of normal bilaterally. Speech discrimination scores at 60 dB were excellent. As part of a screening for retrocochlear disorder speech discrimination was reassessed at high intensity (PI-PB function) and was unchanged on the right but revealed positive retrocochlear signs on the left.

Figure 6–22. Case RJT. ABR at 80 dB nHL revealed bilateral abnormalities. Right Wave V was markedly delayed. Left I-III conduction time was significantly greater than 2.0 msec and therefore was also abnormal. See text.

Figure 6–23. Case RJT. Repeat testing at higher intensity did not improve the ABR response. (See Fig. 6.22).

recording (Fig. 6–23). These results were consistent with retrocochlear pathology evident on stimulation of either ear.

Comment: As mentioned before, these ABR results outline function and change in function of the auditory system, but they do not identify the disease process. However, in view of the reason for work-up—the family history of bilateral acoustic tumor—these findings suggested the presence of bilateral disease in this young man.

Radiologic Examination: On plain X-rays, the internal auditory canal appeared enlarged on the left but smaller and relatively normal on the right. CT scan of the head with enhancement revealed a small lesion on the left.

The family history, positive ABR findings, and positive CT findings in the left ear heightened suspicion. The physician recommended immediate posterior fossa myelography rather than periodic re-evaluation with CT and audiologic tests; the myelogram might make possible an earlier diagnosis, and conservation of hearing by middle fossa removal of the tumor might then be possible. Contrast material failed to enter the right internal auditory canal, suggesting tumor. A 1-cm neurofibroma was removed from the right side. The tumor on the left side was estimated at 1.5 cm but surgery was deferred indefinitely pending the result of efforts to successfully remove the lesion from the right ear with hearing intact.

Audiologic Follow-up: At 2 weeks postoperative, R.J.T. underwent hearing retest and repeat ABR. Hearing retest revealed only slight loss in comparison to the previous test (Fig. 6–24). ABR (Fig. 6–25) revealed marked recovery toward normal.

Otologic Follow-up: R.J.T. was advised to return for hearing recheck if any change in hearing was detected. Annual re-evaluation with hearing test, neurotologic examination, and CT scan was also advised. Resection of the left-ear tumor would be attempted when hearing deteriorated beyond useful levels or the tumor enlarged enough to threaten his neurologic well-being.

SUMMARY

The cases presented in this chapter are examples of the applications of ABR, its integration into the test battery, and some suggestions about reporting.

ABR is recommended when documentation of hearing level is required. It can expedite rehabilitation decisions with the hard to test or confirm accuracy or inaccuracy in cases of conflicting data. ABR is also recommended when site-of-lesion evaluation is indicated, either for (1) suspected auditory disorder at the level of the eighth nerve or above; (2) unilateral tinnitus, pain, hearing loss, or other symptoms suggestive of eighth-nerve lesion; or (3) suspected diffuse neurologic disorders where a brainstem disorder is considered.

Figure 6–24. CASE RJT. Audiogram shows slight decrease in the right ear thresholds following middle fossa surgical removal of a small acoustic nerve tumor (neurofibroma).

Figure 6–25. Case RJT. ABR obtained from the right ear after the tumor was removed showed marked improvement. Upper trace is the pre-operative recording. The lower traces were obtained two weeks post-operatively. Latencies post-operatively fall within normal limits.

Because the test is particularly efficient at predicting acoustic nerve and cerebellopontine angle tumors (see Chapter 5), it should be used as part of the evaluation of pathology to rule them out before management begins. This would include Meniere's disease and other unilateral sensory or neural losses. Sudden sensorineural loss is also an important differential category.

It is important to keep in mind the positive and negative aspects of ABR, and to couch it within the rest of the audiologic, otologic, and neurologic workup.

INDEX

ABR, *see* Auditory brainstem response
Acoustic neurilemmoma, 129–131
Acoustic tumors, 30, 85–86, 105–110
  wave V latencies, 86
Action potentials
  cochlea, 22
  latency of, 24
Adaptation, 24
Age, and audiometric brainstem response
    measurements, 58–59
Alcohol, 48
Aneurysms, 34
Anencephaly, 33
Anesthesia, 48–49
Antibiotics, ototoxic, 30, 79–80
Anticonvulsants, 48
Antimicrobials, 48
Arteriosclerosis, 34
Arteriovenous malformations, 34, 121
Artifacts, 47
Astrocytoma, 33, 116–117
Atherosclerosis, 34
Audiogram shape, reconstruction, 84
Auditory brainstem activity, 25
Auditory brainstem response (ABR)
  applications, 5–6
  biological averaging, 37–39
  brain death, 93
  broad band click, 42
  click stimulus, 84
  clinical applications, 75–98
  clinical experiences, 103–150
  coma, 93
  convention of Jewett, 5
  electrodes, 104
  false negatives, 108
  false positives, case study, 140–142
  far field recording, 75
  filtered clicks, 42–43
  high risk infants, 78–79
  history, 1–3

  limitations, 77–78, 108–110
  logon, 43
  methods, 103–104
  neurotologic evaluation, 77–78
  peripheral threshold sensitivity, 76–77
  response reporting, 63–64
  signal averagers, 104
  single cycle PIP, 43
  site of lesion testing, 76, 84–91
  square wave, 42
  stimulus section, 42–43
  during surgery, 94–98
  technical errors, 70–71
  threshold testing, 78–84
  tone PIPS, 43
  troubleshooting, 69–71
Auditory cortex, 20–21
Auditory evoked potentials
  anatomic terminology, 3–4
  classification of, 3–5
  cochlear microphonic, 4
  contingent negative variant, 4
  continuing potentials, 4
  frequency following response, 4
  glossary, 3–5
  latency, 4–5
    early, 4
    fast, 4–5
    late, 5
    middle, 5
  physiologic terminology, 4
  summating potential, 4
  sustained, 4
Auditory nerve, 18
  tumor, case study, 129–131
Auditory pathways, central, 18–21
  auditory cortex, 20–21
  cochlear nucleus, 18–19
  efferent pathways, 21
  inferior colliculus, 20
  lateral lemniscus, 20